THE OFFICIAL PARENT'S SOURCEBOOK

on

INFANTILE SPASMS

JAMES N. PARKER, M.D.
AND PHILIP M. PARKER, PH.D., EDITORS

ICON Health Publications
ICON Group International, Inc.
4370 La Jolla Village Drive, 4th Floor
San Diego, CA 92122 USA

Printed in the United States of America.

Last digit indicates print number: 10 9 8 7 6 4 5 3 2 1

Publisher, Health Care: Philip Parker, Ph.D.
Editor(s): James Parker, M.D., Philip Parker, Ph.D.

Publisher's note: The ideas, procedures, and suggestions contained in this book are not intended as a substitute for consultation with your child's physician. All matters regarding your child's health require medical supervision. As new medical or scientific information becomes available from academic and clinical research, recommended treatments and drug therapies may undergo changes. The authors, editors, and publisher have attempted to make the information in this book up to date and accurate in accord with accepted standards at the time of publication. The authors, editors, and publisher are not responsible for errors or omissions or for consequences from application of the book, and make no warranty, expressed or implied, in regard to the contents of this book. Any practice described in this book should be applied by the reader in accordance with professional standards of care used in regard to the unique circumstances that may apply in each situation, in close consultation with a qualified physician. The reader is advised to always check product information (package inserts) for changes and new information regarding dose and contraindications before administering any drug or pharmacological product. Caution is especially urged when using new or infrequently ordered drugs, herbal remedies, vitamins and supplements, alternative therapies, complementary therapies and medicines, and integrative medical treatments.

Cataloging-in-Publication Data

Parker, James N., 1961-
Parker, Philip M., 1960-

    The Official Parent's Sourcebook on Infantile Spasms: A Revised and Updated Directory for the Internet Age/James N. Parker and Philip M. Parker, editors
              p.   cm.
    Includes bibliographical references, glossary and index.
    ISBN: 0-497-00985-4
    1. Infantile Spasms-Popular works.   I. Title.

Disclaimer

This publication is not intended to be used for the diagnosis or treatment of a health problem or as a substitute for consultation with licensed medical professionals. It is sold with the understanding that the publisher, editors, and authors are not engaging in the rendering of medical, psychological, financial, legal, or other professional services.

References to any entity, product, service, or source of information that may be contained in this publication should not be considered an endorsement, either direct or implied, by the publisher, editors, or authors. ICON Group International, Inc., the editors, or the authors are not responsible for the content of any Web pages nor publications referenced in this publication.

Copyright Notice

Dedication

To the healthcare professionals dedicating their time and efforts to the study of infantile spasms.

Acknowledgements

The collective knowledge generated from academic and applied research summarized in various references has been critical in the creation of this sourcebook which is best viewed as a comprehensive compilation and collection of information prepared by various official agencies which directly or indirectly are dedicated to infantile spasms. All of the *Official Parent's Sourcebooks* draw from various agencies and institutions associated with the United States Department of Health and Human Services, and in particular, the Office of the Secretary of Health and Human Services (OS), the Administration for Children and Families (ACF), the Administration on Aging (AOA), the Agency for Healthcare Research and Quality (AHRQ), the Agency for Toxic Substances and Disease Registry (ATSDR), the Centers for Disease Control and Prevention (CDC), the Food and Drug Administration (FDA), the Healthcare Financing Administration (HCFA), the Health Resources and Services Administration (HRSA), the Indian Health Service (IHS), the institutions of the National Institutes of Health (NIH), the Program Support Center (PSC), and the Substance Abuse and Mental Health Services Administration (SAMHSA). In addition to these sources, information gathered from the National Library of Medicine, the United States Patent Office, the European Union, and their related organizations has been invaluable in the creation of this sourcebook. Some of the work represented was financially supported by the Research and Development Committee at INSEAD. This support is gratefully acknowledged. Finally, special thanks are owed to Tiffany Freeman for her excellent editorial support.

About the Editors

James N. Parker, M.D.

Dr. James N. Parker received his Bachelor of Science degree in Psychobiology from the University of California, Riverside and his M.D. from the University of California, San Diego. In addition to authoring numerous research publications, he has lectured at various academic institutions. Dr. Parker is the medical editor for the *Official Parent's Sourcebook* series published by ICON Health Publications.

Philip M. Parker, Ph.D.

Philip M. Parker is the Eli Lilly Chair Professor of Innovation, Business and Society at INSEAD (Fontainebleau, France and Singapore). Dr. Parker has also been Professor at the University of California, San Diego and has taught courses at Harvard University, the Hong Kong University of Science and Technology, the Massachusetts Institute of Technology, Stanford University, and UCLA. Dr. Parker is the associate editor for the *Official Parent's Sourcebook* series published by ICON Health Publications.

About ICON Health Publications

In addition to infantile spasms, *Official Parent's Sourcebooks* are available for the following related topics:

- The Official Patient's Sourcebook on Alternating Hemiplegia
- The Official Patient's Sourcebook on Angelman Syndrome
- The Official Patient's Sourcebook on Ataxia Telangiectasia
- The Official Patient's Sourcebook on Brachial Plexus Birth Injuries
- The Official Patient's Sourcebook on Febrile Seizures
- The Official Patient's Sourcebook on Kearns Sayre
- The Official Patient's Sourcebook on Klippel Feil
- The Official Patient's Sourcebook on Lennox Gastaut
- The Official Patient's Sourcebook on Melkersson Rosenthal Syndrome
- The Official Patient's Sourcebook on Mitochondrial Myopathies
- The Official Patient's Sourcebook on Monomelic Amyotrophy
- The Official Patient's Sourcebook on Ohtahara Syndrome
- The Official Patient's Sourcebook on Rasmussen Encephalitis
- The Official Patient's Sourcebook on Reye Syndrome
- The Official Patient's Sourcebook on Sturge Weber
- The Official Patient's Sourcebook on Subacute Sclerosing Panencephalitis
- The Official Patient's Sourcebook on Sydenham Chorea

To discover more about ICON Health Publications, simply check with your preferred online booksellers, including Barnes&Noble.com and Amazon.com which currently carry all of our titles. Or, feel free to contact us directly for bulk purchases or institutional discounts:

ICON Group International, Inc.
4370 La Jolla Village Drive, Fourth Floor
San Diego, CA 92122 USA
Fax: 858-546-4341
Web site: **www.icongrouponline.com/health**

Table of Contents

INTRODUCTION 1
   Overview *1*
   Organization *3*
   Scope *3*
   Moving Forward...*4*

PART I: THE ESSENTIALS 7

CHAPTER 1. THE ESSENTIALS ON INFANTILE SPASMS: GUIDELINES....9
   Overview *9*
   What Are Infantile Spasms? *10*
   Is There Any Treatment? *11*
   What Is the Prognosis?...*11*
   What Research Is Being Done? *11*
   Selected References *12*
   For More Information..*12*
   More Guideline Sources *13*
   Vocabulary Builder *15*

CHAPTER 2. SEEKING GUIDANCE...............................17
   Overview *17*
   Finding Associations *17*
   Finding Doctors...*19*
   Finding a Neurologist *20*
   Selecting Your Child's Doctor.......................................*20*
   Working with Your Child's Doctor *21*
   Broader Health-Related Resources *22*
   Vocabulary Builder *22*

CHAPTER 3. CLINICAL TRIALS AND INFANTILE SPASMS 23
   Overview *23*
   Recent Trials on Infantile Spasms................................*26*
   Benefits and Risks..*28*
   Keeping Current on Clinical Trials................................*31*
   General References..*32*
   Vocabulary Builder *32*

PART II: ADDITIONAL RESOURCES AND ADVANCED MATERIAL..35

CHAPTER 4. STUDIES ON INFANTILE SPASMS 37
   Overview *37*
   Federally Funded Research on Infantile Spasms...........*37*
   The National Library of Medicine: PubMed *43*
   Vocabulary Builder..*97*

CHAPTER 5. PATENTS ON INFANTILE SPASMS 101
  Overview 101
  Patent Applications on Infantile Spasms 102
  Keeping Current 103

CHAPTER 6. BOOKS ON INFANTILE SPASMS 105
  Overview 105
  Book Summaries: Online Booksellers 105
  Chapters on Infantile Spasms 106
  General Home References 106

CHAPTER 7. PERIODICALS AND NEWS ON INFANTILE SPASMS 109
  Overview 109
  News Services and Press Releases 109
  Academic Periodicals covering Infantile Spasms 111

CHAPTER 8. PHYSICIAN GUIDELINES AND DATABASES 119
  Overview 119
  NIH Guidelines 119
  NIH Databases 120
  Other Commercial Databases 124

PART III. APPENDICES 125

APPENDIX A. RESEARCHING YOUR CHILD'S MEDICATIONS 127
  Overview 127
  Your Child's Medications: The Basics 127
  Learning More about Your Child's Medications 129
  Commercial Databases 130
  Researching Orphan Drugs 131
  Contraindications and Interactions (Hidden Dangers) 133
  A Final Warning 134
  General References 134
  Vocabulary Builder 135

APPENDIX B. RESEARCHING ALTERNATIVE MEDICINE 137
  Overview 137
  What Is CAM? 137
  What Are the Domains of Alternative Medicine? 138
  Can Alternatives Affect My Child's Treatment? 141
  Additional Web Resources 146
  General References 147
  Vocabulary Builder 148

APPENDIX C. RESEARCHING NUTRITION 149
  Overview 149
  Food and Nutrition: General Principles 149
  Finding Studies on Infantile Spasms 154
  Federal Resources on Nutrition 159

Additional Web Resources 160
Vocabulary Builder 160
APPENDIX D. FINDING MEDICAL LIBRARIES 161
Overview 161
Preparation 161
Finding a Local Medical Library 162
Medical Libraries in the U.S. and Canada 162
APPENDIX E. SEIZURES AND EPILEPSY: HOPE THROUGH RESEARCH
 169
Overview 169
What Causes Epilepsy? 171
What Are the Different Kinds of Seizures? 174
What Are the Different Kinds of Epilepsy? 176
When Are Seizures Not Epilepsy? 179
How Is Epilepsy Diagnosed? 181
Can Epilepsy Be Prevented? 183
How Can Epilepsy Be Treated? 183
How Does Epilepsy Affect Daily Life? 191
Are There Special Risks Associated with Epilepsy? 195
What Research Is Being Done on Epilepsy? 196
How Can I Help Research on Epilepsy? 198
What to Do If You See Someone Having a Seizure 200
Conclusion 201
Information Resources 202

ONLINE GLOSSARIES 207
Online Dictionary Directories 208

INFANTILE SPASMS GLOSSARY 209
General Dictionaries and Glossaries 213

INDEX 217

INTRODUCTION

Overview

Dr. C. Everett Koop, former U.S. Surgeon General, once said, "The best prescription is knowledge."[1] The Agency for Healthcare Research and Quality (AHRQ) of the National Institutes of Health (NIH) echoes this view and recommends that all parents incorporate education into the treatment process. According to the AHRQ:

> Finding out more about your [child's] condition is a good place to start. By contacting groups that support your [child's] condition, visiting your local library, and searching on the Internet, you can find good information to help guide your decisions for your [child's] treatment. Some information may be hard to find—especially if you don't know where to look.[2]

As the AHRQ mentions, finding the right information is not an obvious task. Though many physicians and public officials had thought that the emergence of the Internet would do much to assist parents in obtaining reliable information, in March 2001 the National Institutes of Health issued the following warning:

> The number of Web sites offering health-related resources grows every day. Many sites provide valuable information, while others may have information that is unreliable or misleading.[3]

---

[1] Quotation from **http://www.drkoop.com**.
[2] The Agency for Healthcare Research and Quality (AHRQ):
http://www.ahcpr.gov/consumer/diaginfo.htm.
[3] From the NIH, National Cancer Institute (NCI):
http://cancertrials.nci.nih.gov/beyond/evaluating.html.

Since the late 1990s, physicians have seen a general increase in parent Internet usage rates. Parents frequently enter their children's doctor's offices with printed Web pages of home remedies in the guise of latest medical research. This scenario is so common that doctors often spend more time dispelling misleading information than guiding children through sound therapies. *The Official Parent's Sourcebook on Infantile Spasms* has been created for parents who have decided to make education and research an integral part of the treatment process. The pages that follow will tell you where and how to look for information covering virtually all topics related to infantile spasms, from the essentials to the most advanced areas of research.

The title of this book includes the word "official." This reflects the fact that the sourcebook draws from public, academic, government, and peer-reviewed research. Selected readings from various agencies are reproduced to give you some of the latest official information available to date on infantile spasms.

Given parents' increasing sophistication in using the Internet, abundant references to reliable Internet-based resources are provided throughout this sourcebook. Where possible, guidance is provided on how to obtain free-of-charge, primary research results as well as more detailed information via the Internet. E-book and electronic versions of this sourcebook are fully interactive with each of the Internet sites mentioned (clicking on a hyperlink automatically opens your browser to the site indicated). Hard copy users of this sourcebook can type cited Web addresses directly into their browsers to obtain access to the corresponding sites. Since we are working with ICON Health Publications, hard copy *Sourcebooks* are frequently updated and printed on demand to ensure that the information provided is current.

In addition to extensive references accessible via the Internet, every chapter presents a "Vocabulary Builder." Many health guides offer glossaries of technical or uncommon terms in an appendix. In editing this sourcebook, we have decided to place a smaller glossary within each chapter that covers terms used in that chapter. Given the technical nature of some chapters, you may need to revisit many sections. Building one's vocabulary of medical terms in such a gradual manner has been shown to improve the learning process.

We must emphasize that no sourcebook on infantile spasms should affirm that a specific diagnostic procedure or treatment discussed in a research study, patent, or doctoral dissertation is "correct" or your child's best option. This sourcebook is no exception. Each child is unique. Deciding on appropriate options is always up to parents in consultation with their children's physicians and healthcare providers.

Organization

This sourcebook is organized into three parts. Part I explores basic techniques to researching infantile spasms (e.g. finding guidelines on diagnosis, treatments, and prognosis), followed by a number of topics, including information on how to get in touch with organizations, associations, or other parent networks dedicated to infantile spasms. It also gives you sources of information that can help you find a doctor in your local area specializing in treating infantile spasms. Collectively, the material presented in Part I is a complete primer on basic research topics for infantile spasms.

Part II moves on to advanced research dedicated to infantile spasms. Part II is intended for those willing to invest many hours of hard work and study. It is here that we direct you to the latest scientific and applied research on infantile spasms. When possible, contact names, links via the Internet, and summaries are provided. It is in Part II where the vocabulary process becomes important as authors publishing advanced research frequently use highly specialized language. In general, every attempt is made to recommend "free-to-use" options.

Part III provides appendices of useful background reading covering infantile spasms or related disorders. The appendices are dedicated to more pragmatic issues facing parents. Accessing materials via medical libraries may be the only option for some parents, so a guide is provided for finding local medical libraries which are open to the public. Part III, therefore, focuses on advice that goes beyond the biological and scientific issues facing children with infantile spasms and their families.

Scope

While this sourcebook covers infantile spasms, doctors, research publications, and specialists may refer to your child's condition using a variety of terms. Therefore, you should understand that infantile spasms is often considered a synonym or a condition closely related to the following:

- Generalized Flexion Epilepsy
- Infantile Epileptic Encephalopathy

- Infantile Myoclonic Encephalopathy
- Infantile Spasms
- Jackknife Convulsion
- Massive Myoclonia
- Salaam Spasms

In addition to synonyms and related conditions, physicians may refer to infantile spasms using certain coding systems. The International Classification of Diseases, 9th Revision, Clinical Modification (ICD-9-CM) is the most commonly used system of classification for the world's illnesses. Your physician may use this coding system as an administrative or tracking tool. The following classification is commonly used for infantile spasms:[4]

- 345.6 infantile spasms

For the purposes of this sourcebook, we have attempted to be as inclusive as possible, looking for official information for all of the synonyms relevant to infantile spasms. You may find it useful to refer to synonyms when accessing databases or interacting with healthcare professionals and medical librarians.

Moving Forward

Since the 1980s, the world has seen a proliferation of healthcare guides covering most illnesses. Some are written by parents, patients, or their family members. These generally take a layperson's approach to understanding and coping with an illness or disorder. They can be uplifting, encouraging, and highly supportive. Other guides are authored by physicians or other healthcare providers who have a more clinical outlook. Each of these two styles of guide has its purpose and can be quite useful.

As editors, we have chosen a third route. We have chosen to expose you to as many sources of official and peer-reviewed information as practical, for the purpose of educating you about basic and advanced knowledge as recognized by medical science today. You can think of this sourcebook as your personal Internet age reference librarian.

---

[4] This list is based on the official version of the World Health Organization's 9th Revision, International Classification of Diseases (ICD-9). According to the National Technical Information Service, "ICD-9CM extensions, interpretations, modifications, addenda, or errata other than those approved by the U.S. Public Health Service and the Health Care Financing Administration are not to be considered official and should not be utilized. Continuous maintenance of the ICD-9-CM is the responsibility of the federal government."

Why "Internet age"? When their child has been diagnosed with infantile spasms, parents will often log on to the Internet, type words into a search engine, and receive several Web site listings which are mostly irrelevant or redundant. Parents are left to wonder where the relevant information is, and how to obtain it. Since only the smallest fraction of information dealing with infantile spasms is even indexed in search engines, a non-systematic approach often leads to frustration and disappointment. With this sourcebook, we hope to direct you to the information you need that you would not likely find using popular Web directories. Beyond Web listings, in many cases we will reproduce brief summaries or abstracts of available reference materials. These abstracts often contain distilled information on topics of discussion.

While we focus on the more scientific aspects of infantile spasms, there is, of course, the emotional side to consider. Later in the sourcebook, we provide a chapter dedicated to helping you find parent groups and associations that can provide additional support beyond research produced by medical science. We hope that the choices we have made give you and your child the most options in moving forward. In this way, we wish you the best in your efforts to incorporate this educational approach into your child's treatment plan.

The Editors

PART I: THE ESSENTIALS

ABOUT PART I

Part I has been edited to give you access to what we feel are "the essentials" on infantile spasms. The essentials typically include a definition or description of the condition, a discussion of who it affects, the signs or symptoms, tests or diagnostic procedures, and treatments for disease. Your child's doctor or healthcare provider may have already explained the essentials of infantile spasms to you or even given you a pamphlet or brochure describing the condition. Now you are searching for more in-depth information. As editors, we have decided, nevertheless, to include a discussion on where to find essential information that can complement what the doctor has already told you. In this section we recommend a process, not a particular Web site or reference book. The process ensures that, as you search the Web, you gain background information in such a way as to maximize your understanding.

CHAPTER 1. THE ESSENTIALS ON INFANTILE SPASMS: GUIDELINES

Overview

Official agencies, as well as federally funded institutions supported by national grants, frequently publish a variety of guidelines on infantile spasms. These are typically called "Fact Sheets" or "Guidelines." They can take the form of a brochure, information kit, pamphlet, or flyer. Often they are only a few pages in length. The great advantage of guidelines over other sources is that they are often written with the parent in mind. Since new guidelines on infantile spasms can appear at any moment and be published by a number of sources, the best approach to finding guidelines is to systematically scan the Internet-based services that post them.

The National Institutes of Health (NIH)[5]

The National Institutes of Health (NIH) is the first place to search for relatively current guidelines and fact sheets on infantile spasms. Originally founded in 1887, the NIH is one of the world's foremost medical research centers and the federal focal point for medical research in the United States. At any given time, the NIH supports some 35,000 research grants at universities, medical schools, and other research and training institutions, both nationally and internationally. The rosters of those who have conducted research or who have received NIH support over the years include the world's most illustrious scientists and physicians. Among them are 97 scientists who have won the Nobel Prize for achievement in medicine.

---

[5] Adapted from the NIH: **http://www.nih.gov/about/NIHoverview.html**.

There is no guarantee that any one Institute will have a guideline on a specific medical condition, though the National Institutes of Health collectively publish over 600 guidelines for both common and rare disorders. The best way to access NIH guidelines is via the Internet. Although the NIH is organized into many different Institutes and Offices, the following is a list of key Web sites where you are most likely to find NIH clinical guidelines and publications dealing with infantile spasms and associated conditions:

- Office of the Director (OD); guidelines consolidated across agencies available at **http://www.nih.gov/health/consumer/conkey.htm**

- National Library of Medicine (NLM); extensive encyclopedia (A.D.A.M., Inc.) with guidelines available at **http://www.nlm.nih.gov/medlineplus/healthtopics.html**

- National Institute of Neurological Disorders and Stroke (NINDS); **http://www.ninds.nih.gov/health_and_medical/disorder_index.htm**

Among the above, the National Institute of Neurological Disorders and Stroke (NINDS) is particularly noteworthy. The mission of the NINDS is to reduce the burden of neurological disease—a burden borne by every age group, by every segment of society, by people all over the world.[6] To support this mission, the NINDS conducts, fosters, coordinates, and guides research on the causes, prevention, diagnosis, and treatment of neurological disorders and stroke, and supports basic research in related scientific areas. The following patient guideline was recently published by the NINDS on infantile spasms.

What Are Infantile Spasms?[7]

Infantile spasm (IS) is a specific type of seizure seen in an epilepsy syndrome of infancy and early childhood known as West Syndrome. The onset is predominantly in the first year of life, typically between 3-6 months. The typical pattern of IS is a sudden bending forward and stiffening of the body, arms, and legs; although there can also be arching of the torso. Spasms tend to begin soon after arousal from sleep. Individual spasms typically last for 1 to 5 seconds and occur in clusters, ranging from 2 to 100 spasms at a time. Infants may have dozens of clusters and several hundred spasms per day.

---

[6] This paragraph has been adapted from the NINDS: **http://www.ninds.nih.gov/about_ninds/mission.htm**. "Adapted" signifies that a passage has been reproduced exactly or slightly edited for this book.

[7] Adapted from The National Institute of Neurological Disorders and Stroke (NINDS): **http://www.ninds.nih.gov/health_and_medical/disorders/infantilespasms.htm**.

Infantile spasms usually stop by age 5, but are often replaced by other seizure types. West Syndrome is characterized by infantile spasms, hypsarrhythmia (abnormal, chaotic brain wave patterns), and mental retardation. Other neurological disorders, such as cerebral palsy, may be seen in 30-50% of those with IS.

Is There Any Treatment?

Treatment with corticosteroids such as ACTH (adrenocorticotrophic hormone) and prednisone is standard, despite the risk of serious side effects. Newer antiepileptic medications, such as vigabatrin (currently not approved for use in the US) have shown some efficacy. A small minority of children has secondarily generalized spasms as the result of cortical lesions (areas of damaged brain tissue). Removal of these lesions may result in improvement.

What Is the Prognosis?

The prognosis for children with IS is dependent on the underlying causes of the seizures. The intellectual prognosis for children with IS is generally poor because many babies with IS have neurological impairment prior to the onset of spasms. Spasms usually resolve with or without treatment by mid-childhood, but more than half of the children with IS will develop other types of seizures. There appears to be a close relationship between IS and Lennox-Gastaut Syndrome, an epileptic disorder of later childhood.

What Research Is Being Done?

The NINDS supports broad and varied programs of research on epilepsy and other seizure disorders. This research is aimed at discovering new ways to prevent, diagnose, and treat these disorders and, ultimately, to find cures for them. Hopefully, more effective and safer treatments, such as neuroprotective agents, will be developed to treat IS and West Syndrome.

Selected References

Aicardi, J.
Infantile Spasms. In Epilepsy in Children, 2nd edition, Raven Press, New York (1994).

Kolodgie, M.
Home Care Management of the Child With Infantile Spasms. Pediatric Nursing, 20:3; 259, 270-273 (May-June 1994).

Haines, S, and Casto, D.
Treatment of Infantile Spasms. Annals of Pharmacotherapy, 28; 779-791 (June 1994).

Dulac, O, Plovin, P.
Cryptogenic/Idiopathic West Syndrome. In: Dulac, O, Chugani, YD, DallaBernadine, B, eds. Infantile Spasms and West Syndrome. London, WB Saunders, (1994).

Hrachovy, R, and Frost, J.
Severe Encephalopathic Epilepsy in Infants: Infantile Spasms. In Childhood Epilepsy and Its Treatment, Demos, New York, NY, pp. 135-145 (1993).

Bobele, G, and Bodensteiner, J.
Infantile Spasms. Neurologic Clinics, 8:3; 633-645 (August 1990).

Hrachovy, R, and Frost, J.
Infantile Spasms. Pediatric Clinics of North America, 36; 311-329 (1989).

For More Information

For more information, contact:

Epilepsy Foundation
4351 Garden City Drive
Suite 500
Landover, MD 20785-7223
postmaster@efa.org
http://www.epilepsyfoundation.org
Tel: 301-459-3700 / 800-EFA-1000 (332-1000)
Fax: 301-577-2684

National Organization for Rare Disorders (NORD)
P.O. Box 8923
(100 Route 37)
New Fairfield, CT 06812-8923
orphan@rarediseases.org
http://www.rarediseases.org
Tel: 203-746-6518 / 800-999-NORD (6673)
Fax: 203-746-6481

More Guideline Sources

The guideline above on infantile spasms is only one example of the kind of material that you can find online and free of charge. The remainder of this chapter will direct you to other sources which either publish or can help you find additional guidelines on topics related to infantile spasms. Many of the guidelines listed below address topics that may be of particular relevance to your child's specific situation, while certain guidelines will apply to only some children with infantile spasms. Due to space limitations these sources are listed in a concise manner. Do not hesitate to consult the following sources by either using the Internet hyperlink provided, or, in cases where the contact information is provided, contacting the publisher or author directly.

Topic Pages: MEDLINEplus

For parents wishing to go beyond guidelines published by specific Institutes of the NIH, the National Library of Medicine has created a vast and parent-oriented healthcare information portal called MEDLINEplus. Within this Internet-based system are "health topic pages." You can think of a health topic page as a guide to patient guides. To access this system, log on to **http://www.nlm.nih.gov/medlineplus/healthtopics.html**. From there you can either search using the alphabetical index or browse by broad topic areas. Recently, MEDLINEplus listed the following as being relevant to infantile spasms:

Epilepsy
http://www.nlm.nih.gov/medlineplus/epilepsy.html

Brain Diseases
http://www.nlm.nih.gov/medlineplus/braindiseases.html

Degenerative Nerve Diseases
http://www.nlm.nih.gov/medlineplus/degenerativenervediseases.html

Head and Brain Malformations
http://www.nlm.nih.gov/medlineplus/headandbrainmalformations.html

Leukodystrophies
http://www.nlm.nih.gov/medlineplus/leukodystrophies.html

Neurologic Diseases
http://www.nlm.nih.gov/medlineplus/neurologicdiseases.html

Neuromuscular Disorders
http://www.nlm.nih.gov/medlineplus/neuromusculardisorders.html

Sleep Disorders
http://www.nlm.nih.gov/medlineplus/sleepdisorders.html

Tuberous Sclerosis
http://www.nlm.nih.gov/medlineplus/tuberoussclerosis.html

You may also choose to use the search utility provided by MEDLINEplus at the following Web address: **http://www.nlm.nih.gov/medlineplus/**. Simply type a keyword into the search box and click "Search." This utility is similar to the NIH search utility, with the exception that it only includes materials that are linked within the MEDLINEplus system (mostly patient-oriented information). It also has the disadvantage of generating unstructured results. We recommend, therefore, that you use this method only if you have a very targeted search.

The NIH Search Utility

After browsing the references listed at the beginning of this chapter, you may want to explore the NIH search utility. This allows you to search for documents on over 100 selected Web sites that comprise the NIH-WEB-SPACE. Each of these servers is "crawled" and indexed on an ongoing basis. Your search will produce a list of various documents, all of which will relate in some way to infantile spasms. The drawbacks of this approach are that the information is not organized by theme and that the references are often a mix of information for professionals and parents. Nevertheless, a large number of the listed Web sites provide useful background information. We can only recommend this route, therefore, for relatively rare or specific disorders, or when using highly targeted searches. To use the NIH search utility, visit the following Web page: **http://search.nih.gov/index.html**.

Additional Web Sources

A number of Web sites that often link to government sites are available to the public. These can also point you in the direction of essential information. The following is a representative sample:

- AOL: **http://search.aol.com/cat.adp?id=168&layer=&from=subcats**

- Family Village: **http://www.familyvillage.wisc.edu/specific.htm**

- Google:
  http://directory.google.com/Top/Health/Conditions_and_Diseases/

- Med Help International: **http://www.medhelp.org/HealthTopics/A.html**

- Open Directory Project:
  http://dmoz.org/Health/Conditions_and_Diseases/

- Yahoo.com: **http://dir.yahoo.com/Health/Diseases_and_Conditions/**

- WebMD®Health: **http://my.webmd.com/health_topics**

Vocabulary Builder

The material in this chapter may have contained a number of unfamiliar words. The following Vocabulary Builder introduces you to terms used in this chapter that have not been covered in the previous chapter:

Impairment: In the context of health experience, an impairment is any loss or abnormality of psychological, physiological, or anatomical structure or function. [NIH]

Infancy: The period of complete dependency prior to the acquisition of competence in walking, talking, and self-feeding. [NIH]

Nerve: A cordlike structure of nervous tissue that connects parts of the nervous system with other tissues of the body and conveys nervous impulses to, or away from, these tissues. [NIH]

Palsy: Disease of the peripheral nervous system occurring usually after many years of increased lead absorption. [NIH]

Tuberous Sclerosis: A rare congenital disease in which the essential pathology is the appearance of multiple tumors in the cerebrum and in other organs, such as the heart or kidneys. [NIH]

CHAPTER 2. SEEKING GUIDANCE

Overview

Some parents are comforted by the knowledge that a number of organizations dedicate their resources to helping people with infantile spasms. These associations can become invaluable sources of information and advice. Many associations offer parent support, financial assistance, and other important services. Furthermore, healthcare research has shown that support groups often help people to better cope with their conditions.[8] In addition to support groups, your child's physician can be a valuable source of guidance and support.

In this chapter, we direct you to resources that can help you find parent organizations and medical specialists. We begin by describing how to find associations and parent groups that can help you better understand and cope with your child's condition. The chapter ends with a discussion on how to find a doctor that is right for your child.

Finding Associations

There are a several Internet directories that provide lists of medical associations with information on or resources relating to infantile spasms. By consulting all of associations listed in this chapter, you will have nearly exhausted all sources for patient associations concerned with infantile spasms.

---

[8] Churches, synagogues, and other houses of worship might also have groups that can offer you the social support you need.

The National Health Information Center (NHIC)

The National Health Information Center (NHIC) offers a free referral service to help people find organizations that provide information about infantile spasms. For more information, see the NHIC's Web site at **http://www.health.gov/NHIC/** or contact an information specialist by calling 1-800-336-4797.

DIRLINE

A comprehensive source of information on associations is the DIRLINE database maintained by the National Library of Medicine. The database comprises some 10,000 records of organizations, research centers, and government institutes and associations which primarily focus on health and biomedicine. DIRLINE is available via the Internet at the following Web site: **http://dirline.nlm.nih.gov**. Simply type in "infantile spasms" (or a synonym) or the name of a topic, and the site will list information contained in the database on all relevant organizations.

The Combined Health Information Database

Another comprehensive source of information on healthcare associations is the Combined Health Information Database. Using the "Detailed Search" option, you will need to limit your search to "Organizations" and "infantile spasms". Type the following hyperlink into your Web browser: **http://chid.nih.gov/detail/detail.html**. To find associations, use the drop boxes at the bottom of the search page where "You may refine your search by." For publication date, select "All Years." Then, select your preferred language and the format option "Organization Resource Sheet." By making these selections and typing in "infantile spasms" (or synonyms) into the "For these words:" box, you will only receive results on organizations dealing with infantile spasms. You should check back periodically with this database since it is updated every 3 months.

The National Organization for Rare Disorders, Inc.

The National Organization for Rare Disorders, Inc. has prepared a Web site that provides, at no charge, lists of associations organized by specific medical conditions. You can access this database at the following Web site:

http://www.rarediseases.org/search/orgsearch.html.   Type   "infantile spasms" (or a synonym) in the search box, and click "Submit Query."

Online Support Groups

In addition to support groups, commercial Internet service providers offer forums and chat rooms to discuss different illnesses and conditions. WebMD®, for example, offers such a service at its Web site: **http://boards.webmd.com/roundtable**. These online communities can help you connect with a network of people whose concerns are similar to yours. Online support groups are places where people can talk informally. If you read about a novel approach, consult with your child's doctor or other healthcare providers, as the treatments or discoveries you hear about may not be scientifically proven to be safe and effective.

Finding Doctors

All parents must go through the process of selecting a physician for their children with infantile spasms. While this process will vary, the Agency for Healthcare Research and Quality makes a number of suggestions, including the following:[9]

- If your child is in a managed care plan, check the plan's list of doctors first.

- Ask doctors or other health professionals who work with doctors, such as hospital nurses, for referrals.

- Call a hospital's doctor referral service, but keep in mind that these services usually refer you to doctors on staff at that particular hospital. The services do not have information on the quality of care that these doctors provide.

- Some local medical societies offer lists of member doctors. Again, these lists do not have information on the quality of care that these doctors provide.

Additional steps you can take to locate doctors include the following:

- Check with the associations listed earlier in this chapter.

---

[9] This section has been adapted from the AHRQ:
www.ahrq.gov/consumer/qntascii/qntdr.htm.

- Information on doctors in some states is available on the Internet at **http://www.docboard.org**. This Web site is run by "Administrators in Medicine," a group of state medical board directors.

- The American Board of Medical Specialties can tell you if your child's doctor is board certified. "Certified" means that the doctor has completed a training program in a specialty and has passed an exam, or "board," to assess his or her knowledge, skills, and experience to provide quality patient care in that specialty. Primary care doctors may also be certified as specialists. The AMBS Web site is located at **http://www.abms.org/newsearch.asp**.[10] You can also contact the ABMS by phone at 1-866-ASK-ABMS.

- You can call the American Medical Association (AMA) at 800-665-2882 for information on training, specialties, and board certification for many licensed doctors in the United States. This information also can be found in "Physician Select" at the AMA's Web site: **http://www.ama-assn.org/aps/amahg.htm**.

Finding a Neurologist

The American Academy of Neurology allows you to search for member neurologists by name or location. To use this service, go to **http://www.aan.com/**, select "Find a Neurologist" from the toolbar. Enter your search criteria, and click "Search." To find out more information on a particular neurologist, click on the physician's name.

If the previous sources did not meet your needs, you may want to log on to the Web site of the National Organization for Rare Disorders (NORD) at **http://www.rarediseases.org/**. NORD maintains a database of doctors with expertise in various rare diseases. The Metabolic Information Network (MIN), 800-945-2188, also maintains a database of physicians with expertise in various metabolic diseases.

Selecting Your Child's Doctor[11]

When you have compiled a list of prospective doctors, call each of their offices. First, ask if the doctor accepts your child's health insurance plan and

---

[10] While board certification is a good measure of a doctor's knowledge, it is possible to receive quality care from doctors who are not board certified.
[11] This section has been adapted from the AHRQ: **www.ahrq.gov/consumer/qntascii/qntdr.htm**.

if he or she is taking new patients. If the doctor is not covered by your child's plan, ask yourself if you are prepared to pay the extra costs. The next step is to schedule a visit with your first choice. During the first visit you will have the opportunity to evaluate your child's doctor and to find out if your child feels comfortable with him or her.

Working with Your Child's Doctor[12]

Research has shown that parents who have good relationships with their children's doctors tend to be more satisfied with their children's care. Here are some tips to help you and your child's doctor become partners:

- You know important things about your child's symptoms and health history. Tell the doctor what you think he or she needs to know.

- Always bring any medications your child is currently taking with you to the appointment, or you can bring a list of your child's medications including dosage and frequency information. Talk about any allergies or reactions your child has had to medications.

- Tell your doctor about any natural or alternative medicines your child is taking.

- Bring other medical information, such as x-ray films, test results, and medical records.

- Ask questions. If you don't, the doctor will assume that you understood everything that was said.

- Write down your questions before the doctor's visit. List the most important ones first to make sure that they are addressed.

- Ask the doctor to draw pictures if you think that this will help you and your child understand.

- Take notes. Some doctors do not mind if you bring a tape recorder to help you remember things, but always ask first.

- Take information home. Ask for written instructions. Your child's doctor may also have brochures and audio and videotapes on infantile spasms.

By following these steps, you will enhance the relationship you and your child have with the physician.

---

[12] This section has been adapted from the AHRQ:
www.ahrq.gov/consumer/qntascii/qntdr.htm.

Broader Health-Related Resources

In addition to the references above, the NIH has set up guidance Web sites that can help parents find healthcare professionals. These include:[13]

- Caregivers:
  http://www.nlm.nih.gov/medlineplus/caregivers.html

- Choosing a Doctor or Healthcare Service:
  http://www.nlm.nih.gov/medlineplus/choosingadoctororhealthcareserv ice.html

- Hospitals and Health Facilities:
  http://www.nlm.nih.gov/medlineplus/healthfacilities.html

Vocabulary Builder

The following vocabulary builder provides definitions of words used in this chapter that have not been defined in previous chapters:

Specialist: In medicine, one who concentrates on 1 special branch of medical science. [NIH]

---

[13] You can access this information at
http://www.nlm.nih.gov/medlineplus/healthsystem.html.

CHAPTER 3. CLINICAL TRIALS AND INFANTILE SPASMS

Overview

Very few medical conditions have a single treatment. The basic treatment guidelines that your child's physician has discussed with you, or those that you have found using the techniques discussed in Chapter 1, may provide you with all that you will require. For some patients, current treatments can be enhanced with new or innovative techniques currently under investigation. In this chapter, we will describe how clinical trials work and show you how to keep informed of trials concerning infantile spasms.

What Is a Clinical Trial?[14]

Clinical trials involve the participation of people in medical research. Most medical research begins with studies in test tubes and on animals. Treatments that show promise in these early studies may then be tried with people. The only sure way to find out whether a new treatment is safe, effective, and better than other treatments for infantile spasms is to try it on patients in a clinical trial.

---

[14] The discussion in this chapter has been adapted from the NIH and the NEI: **http://www.nei.nih.gov/health/clinicaltrials%5Ffacts/index.htm**.

What Kinds of Clinical Trials Are There?

Clinical trials are carried out in three phases:

- **Phase I.** Researchers first conduct Phase I trials with small numbers of patients and healthy volunteers. If the new treatment is a medication, researchers also try to determine how much of it can be given safely.

- **Phase II.** Researchers conduct Phase II trials in small numbers of patients to find out the effect of a new treatment on infantile spasms.

- **Phase III.** Finally, researchers conduct Phase III trials to find out how new treatments for infantile spasms compare with standard treatments already being used. Phase III trials also help to determine if new treatments have any side effects. These trials--which may involve hundreds, perhaps thousands, of people--can also compare new treatments with no treatment.

How Is a Clinical Trial Conducted?

Various organizations support clinical trials at medical centers, hospitals, universities, and doctors' offices across the United States. The "principal investigator" is the researcher in charge of the study at each facility participating in the clinical trial. Most clinical trial researchers are medical doctors, academic researchers, and specialists. The "clinic coordinator" knows all about how the study works and makes all the arrangements for your child's visits.

All doctors and researchers who take part in the study on infantile spasms carefully follow a detailed treatment plan called a protocol. This plan fully explains how the doctors will treat your child in the study. The "protocol" ensures that all patients are treated in the same way, no matter where they receive care.

Clinical trials are controlled. This means that researchers compare the effects of the new treatment with those of the standard treatment. In some cases, when no standard treatment exists, the new treatment is compared with no treatment. Patients who receive the new treatment are in the treatment group. Patients who receive a standard treatment or no treatment are in the "control" group. In some clinical trials, patients in the treatment group get a new medication while those in the control group get a placebo. A placebo is a harmless substance, a "dummy" pill, that has no effect on infantile spasms. In other clinical trials, where a new surgery or device (not a medicine) is being tested, patients in the control group may receive a "sham treatment."

This treatment, like a placebo, has no effect on infantile spasms and will not harm your child.

Researchers assign patients "randomly" to the treatment or control group. This is like flipping a coin to decide which patients are in each group. If you choose to have your child participate in a clinical trial, you will not know which group he or she will be appointed to. The chance of any patient getting the new treatment is about 50 percent. You cannot request that your child receive the new treatment instead of the placebo or "sham" treatment. Often, you will not know until the study is over whether your child has been in the treatment group or the control group. This is called a "masked" study. In some trials, neither doctors nor patients know who is getting which treatment. This is called a "double masked" study. These types of trials help to ensure that the perceptions of the participants or doctors will not affect the study results.

Natural History Studies

Unlike clinical trials in which patient volunteers may receive new treatments, natural history studies provide important information to researchers on how infantile spasms develops over time. A natural history study follows patient volunteers to see how factors such as age, sex, race, or family history might make some people more or less at risk for infantile spasms. A natural history study may also tell researchers if diet, lifestyle, or occupation affects how a medical condition develops and progresses. Results from these studies provide information that helps answer questions such as: How fast will a medical condition usually progress? How bad will the condition become? Will treatment be needed?

What Is Expected of Your Child in a Clinical Trial?

Not everyone can take part in a clinical trial for a specific medical condition. Each study enrolls patients with certain features or eligibility criteria. These criteria may include the type and stage of the condition, as well as, the age and previous treatment history of the patient. You or your child's doctor can contact the sponsoring organization to find out more about specific clinical trials and their eligibility criteria. If you would like your child to participate in a clinical trial, your child's doctor must contact one of the trial's investigators and provide details about his or her diagnosis and medical history.

When participating in a clinical trial, your child may be required to have a number of medical tests. Your child may also need to take medications and/or undergo surgery. Depending upon the treatment and the examination procedure, your child may be required to receive inpatient hospital care. He or she may have to return to the medical facility for follow-up examinations. These exams help find out how well the treatment is working. Follow-up studies can take months or years. However, the success of the clinical trial often depends on learning what happens to patients over a long period of time. Only patients who continue to return for follow-up examinations can provide this important long-term information.

Recent Trials on Infantile Spasms

The National Institutes of Health and other organizations sponsor trials on various medical conditions. Because funding for research goes to the medical areas that show promising research opportunities, it is not possible for the NIH or others to sponsor clinical trials for every medical condition at all times. The following lists recent trials dedicated to infantile spasms.[15] If the trial listed by the NIH is still recruiting, your child may be eligible. If it is no longer recruiting or has been completed, then you can contact the sponsors to learn more about the study and, if published, the results. Further information on the trial is available at the Web site indicated. Please note that some trials may no longer be recruiting patients or are otherwise closed. Before contacting sponsors of a clinical trial, consult with your child's physician who can help you determine if your child might benefit from participation.

- **Metabolic Abnormalities in Children with Epilepsy**

  Condition(s): Generalized Epilepsy; Infantile Spasms; Metabolic Disease; Partial Epilepsy; Seizures

  Study Status: This study is no longer recruiting patients.

  Sponsor(s): National Institute of Neurological Disorders and Stroke (NINDS)

  Purpose - Excerpt: This study is designed to use positron emission tomography to measure brain energy use. Positron Emission Tomography (PET) is a technique used to investigate the functional activity of the brain. The PET technique allows doctors to study the normal processes of the brain (central nervous system) of normal individuals and patients with neurologic illnesses without physical / structural damage to the brain. When a region of the brain is active, it

---

[15] These are listed at **www.ClinicalTrials.gov**.

uses more fuel in the form of oxygen and sugar (glucose). As the brain uses more fuel it produces more waste products, carbon dioxide and water. Blood carries fuel to the brain and waste products away from the brain. As brain activity increases blood flow to and from the area of activity increases also. Researchers can label a sugar with a small radioactive molecule called FDG (fluorodeoxyglucose). As areas of the brain use more sugar the PET scan will detect the FDG and show the areas of the brain that are active. By using this technique researchers hope to answer the following questions; 4. Are changes in brain energy use (metabolism) present early in the course of epilepsy 5. Do changes in brain metabolism match the severity of patient's seizures 6. Do changes in metabolism occur over time or in response to drug therapy

Study Type: Observational

Contact(s): see Web site below

Web Site: http://clinicaltrials.gov/ct/show/NCT00001325

- **Phase II Randomized Study of Early Surgery vs Multiple Sequential Antiepileptic Drug Therapy for Infantile Spasms Refractory to Standard Treatment**

Condition(s): Spasms, Infantile; Epilepsy

Study Status: This study is completed.

Sponsor(s): National Center for Research Resources (NCRR); National Institute of Neurological Disorders and Stroke (NINDS); University of California, Los Angeles

Purpose - Excerpt: Objectives: I. Evaluate the efficacy of surgical resection of an identifiable zone of cortical abnormality versus multiple drug therapy in children with infantile spasms refractory to standard therapy. II. Assess how infantile spasms interfere with development and whether this is partially reversible. III. Determine the predictors of good surgical outcome and whether surgery permanently controls seizures and improves development.

Phase(s): Phase II

Study Type: Interventional

Contact(s): see Web site below

Web Site: http://clinicaltrials.gov/ct/show/NCT00004758

Benefits and Risks[16]

What Are the Benefits of Participating in a Clinical Trial?

If you are considering a clinical trial, it is important to realize that your child's participation can bring many benefits:

- A new treatment could be more effective than the current treatment for infantile spasms. Although only half of the participants in a clinical trial receive the experimental treatment, if the new treatment is proved to be more effective and safer than the current treatment, then those patients who did not receive the new treatment during the clinical trial may be among the first to benefit from it when the study is over.

- If the treatment is effective, then it may improve your child's health.

- Clinical trial patients receive the highest quality of medical care. Experts watch them closely during the study and may continue to follow them after the study is over.

- People who take part in trials contribute to scientific discoveries that may help others with infantile spasms. In cases where certain medical conditions run in families, your child's participation may lead to better care or prevention for you and other family members.

The Informed Consent

Once you agree to have your child take part in a clinical trial, you will be asked to sign an "informed consent." This document explains a clinical trial's risks and benefits, the researcher's expectations of you and your child, and your child's rights as a patient.

What Are the Risks?

Clinical trials may involve risks as well as benefits. Whether or not a new treatment will work cannot be known ahead of time. There is always a chance that a new treatment may not work better than a standard treatment. There is also the possibility that it may be harmful. The treatment your child receives may cause side effects that are serious enough to require medical attention.

---

[16] This section has been adapted from ClinicalTrials.gov, a service of the National Institutes of Health:
http://www.clinicaltrials.gov/ct/gui/c/a1r/info/whatis?JServSessionIdzone_ct=9jmun6f291.

How Is Your Child's Safety Protected?

Clinical trials can raise fears of the unknown. Understanding the safeguards that protect your child can ease some of these fears. Before a clinical trial begins, researchers must get approval from their hospital's Institutional Review Board (IRB), an advisory group that makes sure a clinical trial is designed to protect your child's safety. During a clinical trial, doctors will closely watch your child to see if the treatment is working and if he or she is experiencing any side effects. All the results are carefully recorded and reviewed. In many cases, experts from the Data and Safety Monitoring Committee carefully monitor each clinical trial and can recommend that a study be stopped at any time. Your child will only be asked to participate in a clinical trial as a volunteer with your informed consent.

What Are Your Child's Rights in a Clinical Trial?

If your child is eligible for a clinical trial, you will be given information to help you decide whether or not you want him or her to participate. You and your child have the right to:

- Information on all known risks and benefits of the treatments in the study.
- Know how the researchers plan to carry out the study, for how long, and where.
- Know what is expected of your child.
- Know any costs involved for you or your child's insurance provider.
- Know before any of your child's medical or personal information is shared with other researchers involved in the clinical trial.
- Talk openly with doctors and ask any questions.

After your child joins a clinical trial, you and your child have the right to:

- Leave the study at any time. Participation is strictly voluntary.
- Receive any new information about the new treatment.
- Continue to ask questions and get answers.
- Maintain your child's privacy. Your child's name will not appear in any reports based on the study.
- Know whether your child participated in the treatment group or the control group (once the study has been completed).

What about Costs?

In some clinical trials, the research facility pays for treatment costs and other associated expenses. You or your child's insurance provider may have to pay for costs that are considered standard care. These things may include inpatient hospital care, laboratory and other tests, and medical procedures. You also may need to pay for travel between your home and the clinic. You should find out about costs before committing your child to participation in the trial. If your child has health insurance, find out exactly what it will cover. If your child does not have health insurance, or if your child's insurance policy will not cover care, talk to the clinic staff about other options for covering the costs.

What Questions Should You Ask before Your Child Participates in a Clinical Trial?

Questions you should ask when deciding whether or not to enroll your child in a clinical trial include the following:

- What is the purpose of the clinical trial?
- What are the standard treatments for infantile spasms? Why do researchers think the new treatment may be better? What is likely to happen to my child with or without the new treatment?
- What tests and treatments will my child need? Will my child need surgery? Medication? Hospitalization?
- How long will the treatment last? How often will my child have to come back for follow-up exams?
- What are the treatment's possible benefits to my child's condition? What are the short- and long-term risks? What are the possible side effects?
- Will the treatment be uncomfortable? Will it make my child sick? If so, for how long?
- How will my child's health be monitored?
- Where will my child need to go for the clinical trial?
- How much will it cost to participate in the study? What costs are covered by the study? How much will my child's health insurance cover?
- Who will be in charge of my child's care?
- Will taking part in the study affect my child's daily life?

- How does my child feel about taking part in a clinical trial? Will other family members benefit from my child's contributions to new medical knowledge?

Keeping Current on Clinical Trials

Various government agencies maintain databases on trials. The U.S. National Institutes of Health, through the National Library of Medicine, has developed ClinicalTrials.gov to provide the public and physicians with current information about clinical research across the broadest number of medical conditions.

The site was launched in February 2000 and currently contains approximately 5,700 clinical studies in over 59,000 locations worldwide, with most studies being conducted in the United States. ClinicalTrials.gov receives about 2 million hits per month and hosts approximately 5,400 visitors daily. To access this database, simply go to their Web site (**www.clinicaltrials.gov**) and search by "infantile spasms" (or synonyms).

While ClinicalTrials.gov is the most comprehensive listing of NIH-supported clinical trials available, not all trials are in the database. The database is updated regularly, so clinical trials are continually being added. The following is a list of specialty databases affiliated with the National Institutes of Health that offer additional information on trials:

- For clinical studies at the Warren Grant Magnuson Clinical Center located in Bethesda, Maryland, visit their Web site:
  http://clinicalstudies.info.nih.gov/

- For clinical studies conducted at the Bayview Campus in Baltimore, Maryland, visit their Web site:
  http://www.jhbmc.jhu.edu/studies/index.html

- For trials on neurological disorders and stroke, visit and search the Web site sponsored by the National Institute of Neurological Disorders and Stroke of the NIH:
  http://www.ninds.nih.gov/funding/funding_opportunities.htm#Clinica l_Trials

General References

The following references describe clinical trials and experimental medical research. They have been selected to ensure that they are likely to be available from your local or online bookseller or university medical library. These references are usually written for healthcare professionals, so you may consider consulting with a librarian or bookseller who might recommend a particular reference. The following includes some of the most readily available references (sorted alphabetically by title; hyperlinks provide rankings, information and reviews at Amazon.com):

- **A Guide to Patient Recruitment : Today's Best Practices & Proven Strategies** by Diana L. Anderson; Paperback - 350 pages (2001), CenterWatch, Inc.; ISBN: 1930624115; **http://www.amazon.com/exec/obidos/ASIN/1930624115/icongroupinterna**

- **A Step-By-Step Guide to Clinical Trials** by Marilyn Mulay, R.N., M.S., OCN; Spiral-bound - 143 pages Spiral edition (2001), Jones & Bartlett Pub; ISBN: 0763715697; **http://www.amazon.com/exec/obidos/ASIN/0763715697/icongroupinterna**

- **The CenterWatch Directory of Drugs in Clinical Trials** by CenterWatch; Paperback - 656 pages (2000), CenterWatch, Inc.; ISBN: 0967302935; **http://www.amazon.com/exec/obidos/ASIN/0967302935/icongroupinterna**

- **Extending Medicare Reimbursement in Clinical Trials** by Institute of Medicine Staff (Editor), et al; Paperback 1st edition (2000), National Academy Press; ISBN: 0309068886; **http://www.amazon.com/exec/obidos/ASIN/0309068886/icongroupinterna**

- **Handbook of Clinical Trials** by Marcus Flather (Editor); Paperback (2001), Remedica Pub Ltd; ISBN: 1901346293; **http://www.amazon.com/exec/obidos/ASIN/1901346293/icongroupinterna**

Vocabulary Builder

The following vocabulary builder gives definitions of words used in this chapter that have not been defined in previous chapters:

Consultation: A deliberation between two or more physicians concerning the diagnosis and the proper method of treatment in a case. [NIH]

Protocol: The detailed plan for a clinical trial that states the trial's rationale, purpose, drug or vaccine dosages, length of study, routes of administration, who may participate, and other aspects of trial design. [NIH]

Race: A population within a species which exhibits general similarities within itself, but is both discontinuous and distinct from other populations of that species, though not sufficiently so as to achieve the status of a taxon. [NIH]

PART II: ADDITIONAL RESOURCES AND ADVANCED MATERIAL

ABOUT PART II

In Part II, we introduce you to additional resources and advanced research on infantile spasms. All too often, parents who conduct their own research are overwhelmed by the difficulty in finding and organizing information. The purpose of the following chapters is to provide you an organized and structured format to help you find additional information resources on infantile spasms. In Part II, as in Part I, our objective is not to interpret the latest advances on infantile spasms or render an opinion. Rather, our goal is to give you access to original research and to increase your awareness of sources you may not have already considered. In this way, you will come across the advanced materials often referred to in pamphlets, books, or other general works. Once again, some of this material is technical in nature, so consultation with a professional familiar with infantile spasms is suggested.

CHAPTER 4. STUDIES ON INFANTILE SPASMS

Overview

Every year, academic studies are published on infantile spasms or related conditions. Broadly speaking, there are two types of studies. The first are peer reviewed. Generally, the content of these studies has been reviewed by scientists or physicians. Peer-reviewed studies are typically published in scientific journals and are usually available at medical libraries. The second type of studies is non-peer reviewed. These works include summary articles that do not use or report scientific results. These often appear in the popular press, newsletters, or similar periodicals.

In this chapter, we will show you how to locate peer-reviewed references and studies on infantile spasms. We will begin by discussing research that has been summarized and is free to view by the public via the Internet. We then show you how to generate a bibliography on infantile spasms and teach you how to keep current on new studies as they are published or undertaken by the scientific community.

Federally Funded Research on Infantile Spasms

The U.S. Government supports a variety of research studies relating to infantile spasms and associated conditions. These studies are tracked by the Office of Extramural Research at the National Institutes of Health.[17] CRISP

---

[17] Healthcare projects are funded by the National Institutes of Health (NIH), Substance Abuse and Mental Health Services (SAMHSA), Health Resources and Services Administration (HRSA), Food and Drug Administration (FDA), Centers for Disease Control and Prevention (CDCP), Agency for Healthcare Research and Quality (AHRQ), and Office of Assistant Secretary of Health (OASH).

(Computerized Retrieval of Information on Scientific Projects) is a searchable database of federally funded biomedical research projects conducted at universities, hospitals, and other institutions. Visit CRISP at **http://crisp.cit.nih.gov/crisp/crisp_query.generate_screen**. You can perform targeted searches by various criteria including geography, date, as well as topics related to infantile spasms and related conditions.

For most of the studies, the agencies reporting into CRISP provide summaries or abstracts. As opposed to clinical trial research using patients, many federally funded studies use animals or simulated models to explore infantile spasms and related conditions. In some cases, therefore, it may be difficult to understand how some basic or fundamental research could eventually translate into medical practice. The following sample is typical of the type of information found when searching the CRISP database for infantile spasms:

- **Project Title: 1H AND 31P MRSI FOR EPILEPSY LOCALIZATION**

  Principal Investigator & Institution: Laxer, Kenneth D.; Professor of Clinical Medicine and Neuro; Neurology; University of California San Francisco 500 Parnassus Ave San Francisco, Ca 941222747

  Timing: Fiscal Year 2002; Project Start 01-MAY-1994; Project End 30-JUN-2002

  Summary: The long term goal of this application is to improve the outcome of seizure surgery by better presurgical localization of medically refractory epilepsy using a combination of neuroimaging techniques including magnetic resonance imaging (MRI), 1H and 31P MR spectroscopic imaging (MRSI), and 18F-PET. These techniques will be directed at three groups with medically refractory epilepsy who are being evaluated for seizure surgery (numbers for 5 years): 1)patients with medial temporal lobe epilepsy in whom MRI is non-concordant i.e., MRI shows no abnormality, or an abnormality contralateral to the EEG-defined seizure focus (NC-mTLE, n=75), 2) patients with non-lesional neocortical epilepsy (NE, n=100), and 3) children with **Infantile Spasms** (IS, n=100). NC-mTLE and NE patients frequently require invasive EEG recording, have less than a 50 percent probability of becoming seizure free with surgery, and are often not considered for surgery. Post-operative surgical outcome will be analyzed in relation to the pre-operative neuroimaging findings. Hypotheses: 1) NC-mTLE -Patients with medically refractory mTLE without MRI concordance, who have 1H and 31P MRSI measures concordant with the EEG localization (i.e., lobe and side), will have a significantly better post surgical outcome than patients without MRSI concordance. 2a) NE - NE patients without lesions on MRI, will have 1H and 31P MRSI concordant with the EEG localization (i.e., lobe and side), and this concordance will be greater than that provided by 18FDG-PET. 2b) NE - NE patients, who have 1H and 31P MRSI measures concordant with the EEG localization will have a significantly better post surgical outcome than patients without MRSI concordance. 3a) IS - Children with medically refractory **Infantile Spasms** will have 1H and 31P MRSI concordant with the seizure focus determined by a combination of two or more studies (VET, 18FDG-PET, and/or MRI) and this concordance will be greater than that provided by MRI or 18FDG-PET. 3b) IS - IS children, who have 1H and 31P MRSI concordant with the localization provided by the other clinical and imaging studies will have a significantly better post surgical outcome than patients without such concordance. These studies are expected to lead to improved surgical outcome, and to reduce unnecessary surgery, in patients with intractable epilepsy.

Website: http://crisp.cit.nih.gov/crisp/Crisp_Query.Generate_Screen

- **Project Title: CLINICAL EXPERIENCE AND USE OF VIGABATRIN IN PATIENTS WITH INFANTILE SPASMS**

Principal Investigator & Institution: Mitchell, Wendy G.; Professor; University of Southern California 2250 Alcazar Street, Csc-219 Los Angeles, Ca 90033

Timing: Fiscal Year 2002

Summary: This abstract is not available.

Website: http://crisp.cit.nih.gov/crisp/Crisp_Query.Generate_Screen

- **Project Title: EPILEPTOGENESIS IN A RAT MODEL OF TUBEROUS SCLEROSIS**

Principal Investigator & Institution: Emmi, Adriana; Neurological Surgery; University of Washington Grant & Contract Services Seattle, Wa 98105

Timing: Fiscal Year 2002; Project Start 24-SEP-2001; Project End 31-AUG-2004

Summary: (Applicant's abstract): This proposal, a response to the program announcement for exploratory (R21) grants in pediatric brain disorders, focuses on the issue of epileptogenesis in tuberous sclerosis. Tuberous sclerosis (TS) is an autosomal dominant disorder characterized by the formation of hamartomatous growths in multiple organ systems, including kidney, skin, and brain. Recent studies suggest a TS incidence of 1 in 6,000 live births. The most debilitating of the effects of TS are its nervous system manifestations, including epilepsy and mental retardation. It has been estimated that over 80% of TS patients have epilepsy, often occurring early in development as such difficult-to-control syndromes as **infantile spasms.** While insights into TS have been greatly advanced by our understanding of the underlying genes (TSC1 and TSC2), the connections between TS gene mutations and brain hamartomas (and particularly cortical tubers), and between tubers and seizure development, remain unclear. The absence of an animal model of TS with a CNS tuber and seizure phenotype has made it difficult to study these relationships. In this proposal, we exploit the Eker rat, a TSC2 +/- "carrier", to address two aspects of the tuber/epilepsy complex. First, we will examine the hypothesis that cytologically-abnormal cells characteristic of cortical tubers are a result of homozygous mutations at the TSC2 locus (TSC2 -/-); that is, loss of heterozygosity (LOH) is a critical feature of brain tuber formation, just as it is for tumors in other organs (e.g., kidney). TSC2 -/- cells will be obtained from embryonic CNS tissue (from +/- x +/- Eker crosses) and maintained in culture. Morphological and electrophysiological tools will be used to characterize these cells (vs. TSC2 +/- and +/+ cells). Differentiation of cultured TSC2 -/- neuroblasts will be examined under different culture conditions, their response to experimental challenge (e.g., irradiation, excitotoxicity) determined, and their effects on co-cultured tissue assessed. Second, to test the hypothesis that TSC -/- cells give rise to cortical tubers, cultured cells (containing a fluorescent marker gene) will be transplanted into normal rat brain. Morphological features (e.g., tuber formation, circuitry reorganization) of transplanted cortex, as well as its electrical excitability and the animal's seizure susceptibility, will be determined. These studies, while not yet probing the molecular mechanisms through which TSC2 mutations give rise to structural malformations in the developing animal, will address critical phenomenological cause-effect relationships that will serve as the basis for future mechanistic studies.

Website: http://crisp.cit.nih.gov/crisp/Crisp_Query.Generate_Screen

- **Project Title: NEURAL SUBSTRATES /SOCIOEMOTIONAL DISTURBANCES /DEVELOP.**

Principal Investigator & Institution: Malkova, Ludise; Assistant Professor; Pharmacology; Georgetown University Washington, Dc 20057

Timing: Fiscal Year 2002; Project Start 03-AUG-2001; Project End 31-MAY-2004

Summary: (provided by applicant): The goal of this proposal is to understand how early brain insults influence the short-term and long-term development of cognitive and socioemotional functions. This understanding is vital for the approach to neurodevelopmental disorders such as autism, and at the same time is relevant to an entire spectrum of behavioral disorders that emerge as a result of a host of neurological disturbances in children (epilepsy, cerebral palsy, cortical dysgenesis, etc.). The analysis of human cases and experiments in animals suggest the hypothesis that dysfunction in medial temporal lobes, and the amygdala in particular, is an etiological factor in autism. Therefore the goal of our proposal is to investigate the role of the amygdala and its specific subdivisions for socioemotional behavior and to identify the critical developmental periods and neural triggers for developmental abnormalities in an animal model of autism. The first Specific Aim concentrates on the effects of pharmacologically-induced imbalances in neurotransmission in the amygdala on social interactions in infant animals. Drugs known to either block or enhance GABA-ergic or glutamatergic transmission will be focally infused into specific subdivisions of the amygdala and social interactions in the experimental animals will be observed. The second Specific Aim is to compare the effects of drugs (as obtained in Aim I) with the effects of discrete lesions of subregions of the amygdala, when damaged by axon-sparing excitotoxic lesions, in infant monkeys. The third aim will evaluate the effects of early prolonged seizures, known to disrupt the function of the amygdala and its projection network, on the observed behavioral categories. This aim is directed to the understanding why certain seizure disorders in infants (e.g., infantile spasms) give rise to autism. An important facet of these studies will be the analysis of the extent to which socioemotional disturbances produced by various anatomically site-specific insults are accompanied by impairment in cognitive functions. Well standardized procedures will be used to evaluate various components of socioemotional interactions of infant and juvenile animals in dyads and to assess their emotional reactions to positive and negative stimuli. Cognitive tasks will include concurrent visual objects discrimination and auditory-visual crossmodal associations and memory. The results of the proposed studies will identify specific amygdaloid nuclei critical for regulation of social and emotional interactions and determine the critical stage(s) in development during which amygdala dysfunction (by lesions, drugs or seizures) can lead to long-term socioemotional abnormalities. This information will provide a rationale basis for the design of therapeutic interventions directed at correcting the underlying biological dysfunctions that give rise to autism and related socioemotional disorders.

Website: http://crisp.cit.nih.gov/crisp/Crisp_Query.Generate_Screen

- **Project Title: SURGERY FOR INFANTILE SPASMS CORRELATES OF AUTISTIC DISORDER**

  Principal Investigator & Institution: Caplan, Rochelle; Associate Professor; University of California Los Angeles 10920 Wilshire Blvd., Suite 1200 Los Angeles, Ca 90024

  Timing: Fiscal Year 2002; Project Start 01-AUG-2001; Project End 31-JUL-2002

  Summary: Specific Aims 1. To use MR technology to study neurodevelopmental abnormalities in schizophrenia, as revealed through gyrification patterns and the presence of abnormalities in midline structures such as the thalamus 2. To extend our work defining and quantifying surface anatomy to the development of "flat maps" that will provide additional measures of surface complexity 3. To examine hypothesized anatomic substrates of cognitive dysmetria by measuring specific nodes on the CCTCC (e.g.. areas of prefrontal cortex, cerebellum. and thalamus) 4. To develop methods to parcellate and measure structural characteristics of the prefrontal cortex, using indices of sulca/gyral anatomy thus far developed 5. To develop methods to measure structural characteristics of the cerebellum (including both deep nuclei and surface anatomy) using MR 6. To apply the technique of neural networks to develop reliable and automated measures of neural structures relevant to schizophrenia 7. To examine the relationship between CCTCC abnormalities, symptom patterns, and cognitive performance

  Website: http://crisp.cit.nih.gov/crisp/Crisp_Query.Generate_Screen

- **Project Title: VISUALIZATION OF TEMPORAL PATTERNS OF COMPLEX BRAIN ACTIVITY**

  Principal Investigator & Institution: Simpson, Gregory V.;; University of California Los Angeles 10920 Wilshire Blvd., Suite 1200 Los Angeles, Ca 90024

  Timing: Fiscal Year 2002

  Summary: The proposed study will examine the social communication and neuroanatomical correlates of autistic disorder (i.e., qualitative impairment in social interaction, qualitative impairment in communication. restricted repetitive stereotyped patterns of behavior. interests. and activities) in a cohort of surgically treated children with **infantile spasms.** We will also examine the degree of tuberous sclerosis (TSC)-like changes and cortical dysplasias in the resected brain tissue of these children. and determine its correlation with the diagnosis of autism. Specific Aims 1. We will examine the hypothesis that surgically treated children with **infantile spasms** who meet criteria for autistic disorder have specific social communication deficits (i.e., underutilization of joint attention and social interaction, impaired distribution of positive affect during nonverbal communication) at the 2 year follow-up after surgery compared to those who do not meet criteria for autistic disorder. 2. We will examine the hypothesis that the resected hemisphere of the surgically treated **infantile spasms** patients who meet criteria for autistic disorder has more severe cortical dysplasia with TSC-like lesions than the patients who do not meet criteria for autistic disorder. 3. We will test the hypothesis that, compared to the children who do not meet criteria for autistic disorder, the nonresected hemisphere of the children who meet criteria for autistic disorder will have: a) presurgical FDG hypometabolism of the temporal, parietal, and/or frontal lobes b) postsurgical MRI evidence for increased volume of the nonresected hemisphere and reduced area of cerebellar lobules VI and VII. 4. We will examine hypotheses that an intact remaining hemisphere can support social communication by determining if the postoperative change in specific social communication behaviors are associated with presurgical FDG metabolic patterns.

Website: http://crisp.cit.nih.gov/crisp/Crisp_Query.Generate_Screen

The National Library of Medicine: PubMed

One of the quickest and most comprehensive ways to find academic studies in both English and other languages is to use PubMed, maintained by the National Library of Medicine. The advantage of PubMed over previously mentioned sources is that it covers a greater number of domestic and foreign references. It is also free to the public.[18] If the publisher has a Web site that offers full text of its journals, PubMed will provide links to that site, as well as to sites offering other related data. User registration, a subscription fee, or some other type of fee may be required to access the full text of articles in some journals.

To generate your own bibliography of studies dealing with infantile spasms, simply go to the PubMed Web site at **www.ncbi.nlm.nih.gov/pubmed**. Type "infantile spasms" (or synonyms) into the search box, and click "Go." The

---

[18] PubMed was developed by the National Center for Biotechnology Information (NCBI) at the National Library of Medicine (NLM) at the National Institutes of Health (NIH). The PubMed database was developed in conjunction with publishers of biomedical literature as a search tool for accessing literature citations and linking to full-text journal articles at Web sites of participating publishers. Publishers that participate in PubMed supply NLM with their citations electronically prior to or at the time of publication.

following is the type of output you can expect from PubMed for "infantile spasms" (hyperlinks lead to article summaries):

- **A case of infantile spasms: epileptic apnea as partial seizures at onset.**
  Author(s): Kamei A, Ichinohe S, Ito M, Fujiwara T.
  Source: Brain & Development. 1996 May-June; 18(3): 239-41.
  http://www.ncbi.nlm.nih.gov:80/entrez/query.fcgi?cmd=Retrieve&db=PubMed&list_uids=8836510&dopt=Abstract

- **A long-term follow-up study of 214 children with the syndrome of infantile spasms.**
  Author(s): Riikonen R.
  Source: Neuropediatrics. 1982 February; 13(1): 14-23.
  http://www.ncbi.nlm.nih.gov:80/entrez/query.fcgi?cmd=Retrieve&db=PubMed&list_uids=6281679&dopt=Abstract

- **A patient with infantile spasms and low homovanillic acid levels in cerebrospinal fluid: L-dopa dependent seizures?**
  Author(s): Sugie H, Sugie Y, Kato N, Fukuyama Y.
  Source: European Journal of Pediatrics. 1989 June; 148(7): 667-8.
  http://www.ncbi.nlm.nih.gov:80/entrez/query.fcgi?cmd=Retrieve&db=PubMed&list_uids=2744043&dopt=Abstract

- **A pilot study of topiramate in the treatment of infantile spasms.**
  Author(s): Glauser TA, Clark PO, Strawsburg R.
  Source: Epilepsia. 1998 December; 39(12): 1324-8.
  http://www.ncbi.nlm.nih.gov:80/entrez/query.fcgi?cmd=Retrieve&db=PubMed&list_uids=9860068&dopt=Abstract

- **A prospective study of infantile spasms: clinical and therapeutic correlations.**
  Author(s): Lombroso CT.
  Source: Epilepsia. 1983 April; 24(2): 135-58.
  http://www.ncbi.nlm.nih.gov:80/entrez/query.fcgi?cmd=Retrieve&db=PubMed&list_uids=6299719&dopt=Abstract

- **A retrospective study of spontaneous remission and long-term outcome in patients with infantile spasms.**
  Author(s): Hrachovy RA, Glaze DG, Frost JD Jr.
  Source: Epilepsia. 1991 March-April; 32(2): 212-4.
  http://www.ncbi.nlm.nih.gov:80/entrez/query.fcgi?cmd=Retrieve&db=PubMed&list_uids=1848513&dopt=Abstract

- **A risk-benefit assessment of treatments for infantile spasms.**
  Author(s): Nabbout R.
  Source: Drug Safety : an International Journal of Medical Toxicology and Drug Experience. 2001; 24(11): 813-28. Review.
  http://www.ncbi.nlm.nih.gov:80/entrez/query.fcgi?cmd=Retrieve&db=PubMed&list_uids=11665869&dopt=Abstract

- **A special note on terminology of West syndrome and infantile spasms.**
  Author(s): Fukuyama Y.
  Source: Brain & Development. 2001 November; 23(7): 442.
  http://www.ncbi.nlm.nih.gov:80/entrez/query.fcgi?cmd=Retrieve&db=PubMed&list_uids=11701236&dopt=Abstract

- **ACTH activates rapid eye movement-related phasic inhibition during REM sleep in patients with infantile spasms.**
  Author(s): Kohyama J, Shimohira M, Tanuma N, Hasegawa T, Iwakawa Y.
  Source: Acta Neurologica Scandinavica. 2000 March; 101(3): 145-52.
  http://www.ncbi.nlm.nih.gov:80/entrez/query.fcgi?cmd=Retrieve&db=PubMed&list_uids=10705935&dopt=Abstract

- **ACTH induced adrenal enlargement in infants treated for infantile spasms and acute cerebellar encephalopathy.**
  Author(s): Liebling MS, Starc TJ, McAlister WH, Ruzal-Shapiro CB, Abramson SJ, Berdon WE.
  Source: Pediatric Radiology. 1993; 23(6): 454-6.
  http://www.ncbi.nlm.nih.gov:80/entrez/query.fcgi?cmd=Retrieve&db=PubMed&list_uids=8255650&dopt=Abstract

- **ACTH therapy for infantile spasms: a combination therapy with high-dose pyridoxal phosphate and low-dose ACTH.**
  Author(s): Takuma Y.
  Source: Epilepsia. 1998; 39 Suppl 5: 42-5.
  http://www.ncbi.nlm.nih.gov:80/entrez/query.fcgi?cmd=Retrieve&db=PubMed&list_uids=9737444&dopt=Abstract

- **ACTH therapy in infantile spasms: relationship between dose of ACTH and initial effect or long-term prognosis.**
  Author(s): Ito M, Okuno T, Fujii T, Mutoh K, Oguro K, Shiraishi H, Shirasaka Y, Mikawa H.
  Source: Pediatric Neurology. 1990 July-August; 6(4): 240-4.
  http://www.ncbi.nlm.nih.gov:80/entrez/query.fcgi?cmd=Retrieve&db=PubMed&list_uids=2169750&dopt=Abstract

- **ACTH treatment of infantile spasms: mechanisms of its effects in modulation of neuronal excitability.**
  Author(s): Brunson KL, Avishai-Eliner S, Baram TZ.
  Source: Int Rev Neurobiol. 2002; 49: 185-97. Review.
  http://www.ncbi.nlm.nih.gov:80/entrez/query.fcgi?cmd=Retrieve&db=PubMed&list_uids=12040892&dopt=Abstract

- **ACTH versus vigabatrin therapy in infantile spasms: a retrospective study.**
  Author(s): Cossette P, Riviello JJ, Carmant L.
  Source: Neurology. 1999 May 12; 52(8): 1691-4. Erratum In: Neurology 2000 January 25; 54(2): 539.
  http://www.ncbi.nlm.nih.gov:80/entrez/query.fcgi?cmd=Retrieve&db=PubMed&list_uids=10331702&dopt=Abstract

- **Acute-onset transient hydrocephalus after suspension of ACTH therapy for infantile spasms: a case report.**
  Author(s): Laverda AM, Casara G, Battistella PA, Drigo P.
  Source: Italian Journal of Neurological Sciences. 1984 June; 5(2): 219-22.
  http://www.ncbi.nlm.nih.gov:80/entrez/query.fcgi?cmd=Retrieve&db=PubMed&list_uids=6088422&dopt=Abstract

- **Adrenocortical hyporesponsiveness after treatment with ACTH of infantile spasms.**
  Author(s): Perheentupa J, Riikonen R, Dunkel L, Simell O.
  Source: Archives of Disease in Childhood. 1986 August; 61(8): 750-3.
  http://www.ncbi.nlm.nih.gov:80/entrez/query.fcgi?cmd=Retrieve&db=PubMed&list_uids=3017239&dopt=Abstract

- **Adrenocorticotropic hormone and vigabatrin treatment of children with infantile spasms underlying cerebral palsy.**
  Author(s): Zafeiriou DI, Kontopoulos EE, Tsikoulas IG.
  Source: Brain & Development. 1996 November-December; 18(6): 450-2.
  http://www.ncbi.nlm.nih.gov:80/entrez/query.fcgi?cmd=Retrieve&db=PubMed&list_uids=8980841&dopt=Abstract

- **Adrenocorticotropic hormone controls infantile spasms independently of cortisol stimulation.**
  Author(s): Farwell J, Milstein J, Opheim K, Smith E, Glass S.
  Source: Epilepsia. 1984 October; 25(5): 605-8.
  http://www.ncbi.nlm.nih.gov:80/entrez/query.fcgi?cmd=Retrieve&db=PubMed&list_uids=6090111&dopt=Abstract

- **Adrenocorticotropic hormone therapy for infantile spasms alters pyruvate metabolism in the central nervous system.**
  Author(s): Miyazaki M, Hashimoto T, Yoneda Y, Saijio T, Mori K, Ito M, Kuroda Y.
  Source: Brain & Development. 1998 August; 20(5): 312-8.
  http://www.ncbi.nlm.nih.gov:80/entrez/query.fcgi?cmd=Retrieve&db=PubMed&list_uids=9761001&dopt=Abstract

- **Advances in therapy of infantile spasms. Current knowledge of actions of ACTH and corticosteroids.**
  Author(s): Riikonen R.
  Source: Brain & Development. 1987; 9(4): 409-14. Review.
  http://www.ncbi.nlm.nih.gov:80/entrez/query.fcgi?cmd=Retrieve&db=PubMed&list_uids=2829647&dopt=Abstract

- **Aicardi's syndrome: (agenesis of the corpus callosum, infantile spasms, and ocular anomalies).**
  Author(s): Dinani S, Jancar J.
  Source: J Ment Defic Res. 1984 June; 28 (Pt 2): 143-9.
  http://www.ncbi.nlm.nih.gov:80/entrez/query.fcgi?cmd=Retrieve&db=PubMed&list_uids=6748057&dopt=Abstract

- **An investigation of infantile spasms with normal brain CT images.**
  Author(s): Takahashi H, Ohtsuka C, Saito M, Sato Y, Niijima S, Tada H, Takahashi K.
  Source: Jpn J Psychiatry Neurol. 1990 June; 44(2): 349-50. No Abstract Available.
  http://www.ncbi.nlm.nih.gov:80/entrez/query.fcgi?cmd=Retrieve&db=PubMed&list_uids=2175366&dopt=Abstract

- **An unknown combination of infantile spasms, retinal lesions, facial dysmorphism and limb abnormalities.**
  Author(s): Plomp AS, Reardon W, Benton S, Taylor D, Larcher VF, Sundrum R, Winter RM.
  Source: Clinical Dysmorphology. 2000 July; 9(3): 189-92.
  http://www.ncbi.nlm.nih.gov:80/entrez/query.fcgi?cmd=Retrieve&db=PubMed&list_uids=10955479&dopt=Abstract

- **An unusual case of recovery from infantile spasms.**
  Author(s): Riikonen R.
  Source: Developmental Medicine and Child Neurology. 1984 December; 26(6): 818-21.
  http://www.ncbi.nlm.nih.gov:80/entrez/query.fcgi?cmd=Retrieve&db=PubMed&list_uids=6519364&dopt=Abstract

- **Apparent cerebral atrophic findings on cranial computed tomography in nephrotic children with steroid therapy and in patients of infantile spasms with ACTH therapy.**
  Author(s): Yano E.
  Source: Kurume Med J. 1981; 28(1): 63-77. No Abstract Available.
  http://www.ncbi.nlm.nih.gov:80/entrez/query.fcgi?cmd=Retrieve&db=PubMed&list_uids=6275165&dopt=Abstract

- **Asymmetric and asynchronous infantile spasms.**
  Author(s): Gaily EK, Shewmon DA, Chugani HT, Curran JG.
  Source: Epilepsia. 1995 September; 36(9): 873-82.
  http://www.ncbi.nlm.nih.gov:80/entrez/query.fcgi?cmd=Retrieve&db=PubMed&list_uids=7649126&dopt=Abstract

- **Asymmetric hypsarrhythmia and infantile spasms in west syndrome.**
  Author(s): Donat JF, Lo WD.
  Source: Journal of Child Neurology. 1994 July; 9(3): 290-6.
  http://www.ncbi.nlm.nih.gov:80/entrez/query.fcgi?cmd=Retrieve&db=PubMed&list_uids=7930409&dopt=Abstract

- **Auditory brain stem responses in infantile spasms.**
  Author(s): Kaga K, Marsh RR, Fukuyama Y.
  Source: International Journal of Pediatric Otorhinolaryngology. 1982 March; 4(1): 57-67.
  http://www.ncbi.nlm.nih.gov:80/entrez/query.fcgi?cmd=Retrieve&db=PubMed&list_uids=7095993&dopt=Abstract

- **Autism and infantile spasms in children with tuberous sclerosis.**
  Author(s): Curatolo P, Cusmai R.
  Source: Developmental Medicine and Child Neurology. 1987 August; 29(4): 551.
  http://www.ncbi.nlm.nih.gov:80/entrez/query.fcgi?cmd=Retrieve&db=PubMed&list_uids=3678635&dopt=Abstract

- **Autosomal recessive polymicrogyria with infantile spasms and limb deformities.**
  Author(s): Ciardo F, Zamponi N, Specchio N, Parmeggiani L, Guerrini R.
  Source: Neuropediatrics. 2001 December; 32(6): 325-9.
  http://www.ncbi.nlm.nih.gov:80/entrez/query.fcgi?cmd=Retrieve&db=PubMed&list_uids=11870589&dopt=Abstract

- **BAEPs in infantile spasms.**
  Author(s): Curatolo P, Cardona F, Cusmai R.
  Source: Brain & Development. 1989; 11(5): 347-8.
  http://www.ncbi.nlm.nih.gov:80/entrez/query.fcgi?cmd=Retrieve&db=PubMed&list_uids=2817301&dopt=Abstract

- **Benign myoclonus of early infancy or benign non-epileptic infantile spasms.**
  Author(s): Dravet C, Giraud N, Bureau M, Roger J, Gobbi G, Dalla Bernardina B.
  Source: Neuropediatrics. 1986 February; 17(1): 33-8.
  http://www.ncbi.nlm.nih.gov:80/entrez/query.fcgi?cmd=Retrieve&db=PubMed&list_uids=3960282&dopt=Abstract

- **Brain malformations, epilepsy, and infantile spasms.**
  Author(s): Ross ME.
  Source: Int Rev Neurobiol. 2002; 49: 333-52. Review.
  http://www.ncbi.nlm.nih.gov:80/entrez/query.fcgi?cmd=Retrieve&db=PubMed&list_uids=12040900&dopt=Abstract

- **Brain maturational aspects relevant to pathophysiology of infantile spasms.**
  Author(s): Avanzini G, Panzica F, Franceschetti S.
  Source: Int Rev Neurobiol. 2002; 49: 353-65. Review.
  http://www.ncbi.nlm.nih.gov:80/entrez/query.fcgi?cmd=Retrieve&db=PubMed&list_uids=12040901&dopt=Abstract

- **Brain tumors associated with infantile spasms.**
  Author(s): Asanuma H, Wakai S, Tanaka T, Chiba S.
  Source: Pediatric Neurology. 1995 May; 12(4): 361-4.
  http://www.ncbi.nlm.nih.gov:80/entrez/query.fcgi?cmd=Retrieve&db=PubMed&list_uids=7546012&dopt=Abstract

- **Brain-adrenal axis hormones are altered in the CSF of infants with massive infantile spasms.**
  Author(s): Baram TZ, Mitchell WG, Snead OC 3rd, Horton EJ, Saito M.
  Source: Neurology. 1992 June; 42(6): 1171-5.
  http://www.ncbi.nlm.nih.gov:80/entrez/query.fcgi?cmd=Retrieve&db=PubMed&list_uids=1318521&dopt=Abstract

- **Brainstem involvement in infantile spasms: a study employing brainstem evoked potentials and magnetic resonance imaging.**
  Author(s): Miyazaki M, Hashimoto T, Tayama M, Kuroda Y.
  Source: Neuropediatrics. 1993 June; 24(3): 126-30.
  http://www.ncbi.nlm.nih.gov:80/entrez/query.fcgi?cmd=Retrieve&db=PubMed&list_uids=8395028&dopt=Abstract

- **Brainstem tumor with infantile spasms.**
  Author(s): Aktan G, Simsek A, Aysun S.
  Source: Journal of Child Neurology. 1997 February; 12(2): 152-4.
  http://www.ncbi.nlm.nih.gov:80/entrez/query.fcgi?cmd=Retrieve&db=PubMed&list_uids=9075029&dopt=Abstract

- **Brief atonia associated with electroencephalographic paroxysm in an infant with infantile spasms.**
  Author(s): Hakamada S, Watanabe K, Hara K, Miyazaki S.
  Source: Epilepsia. 1981 June; 22(3): 285-8.
  http://www.ncbi.nlm.nih.gov:80/entrez/query.fcgi?cmd=Retrieve&db=PubMed&list_uids=6786865&dopt=Abstract

- **Can barbiturate anaesthesia cure infantile spasms?**
  Author(s): Riikonen R, Santavuori P, Meretoja O, Sainio K, Neuvonen PJ, Tokola RA.
  Source: Brain & Development. 1988; 10(5): 300-4.
  http://www.ncbi.nlm.nih.gov:80/entrez/query.fcgi?cmd=Retrieve&db=PubMed&list_uids=3239696&dopt=Abstract

- **Carbamazepine and benzodiazepines in combination--a possibility to improve the efficacy of treatment of patients with 'intractable' infantile spasms?**
  Author(s): Tatzer E, Groh C, Muller R, Lischka A.
  Source: Brain & Development. 1987; 9(4): 415-7.
  http://www.ncbi.nlm.nih.gov:80/entrez/query.fcgi?cmd=Retrieve&db=PubMed&list_uids=3434716&dopt=Abstract

- **Cerebral malformation in a child with profound psychomotor retardation and infantile spasms.**
  Author(s): Mizuguchi M, Itoh M, Takashima S.
  Source: Neuropathology : Official Journal of the Japanese Society of Neuropathology. 2001 December; 21(4): 333-5.
  http://www.ncbi.nlm.nih.gov:80/entrez/query.fcgi?cmd=Retrieve&db=PubMed&list_uids=11837541&dopt=Abstract

- **Cerebrospinal fluid corticotropin and cortisol are reduced in infantile spasms.**
  Author(s): Baram TZ, Mitchell WG, Hanson RA, Snead OC 3rd, Horton EJ.
  Source: Pediatric Neurology. 1995 September; 13(2): 108-10.
  http://www.ncbi.nlm.nih.gov:80/entrez/query.fcgi?cmd=Retrieve&db=PubMed&list_uids=8534274&dopt=Abstract

- **Cerebrospinal fluid GABA levels in children with infantile spasms.**
  Author(s): Ito M, Mikawa H, Taniguchi T.
  Source: Neurology. 1984 February; 34(2): 235-8.
  http://www.ncbi.nlm.nih.gov:80/entrez/query.fcgi?cmd=Retrieve&db=PubMed&list_uids=6320056&dopt=Abstract

- **Cerebrospinal fluid monoamine metabolites in patients with infantile spasms.**
  Author(s): Silverstein F, Johnston MV.
  Source: Neurology. 1984 January; 34(1): 102-5.
  http://www.ncbi.nlm.nih.gov:80/entrez/query.fcgi?cmd=Retrieve&db=PubMed&list_uids=6197678&dopt=Abstract

- **Changes in CSF neurotransmitters in infantile spasms.**
  Author(s): Langlais PJ, Wardlow ML, Yamamoto H.
  Source: Pediatric Neurology. 1991 November-December; 7(6): 440-5.
  http://www.ncbi.nlm.nih.gov:80/entrez/query.fcgi?cmd=Retrieve&db=PubMed&list_uids=1724602&dopt=Abstract

- **Choroid plexus papilloma and infantile spasms.**
  Author(s): Branch CE, Dyken PR.
  Source: Annals of Neurology. 1979 March; 5(3): 302-4.
  http://www.ncbi.nlm.nih.gov:80/entrez/query.fcgi?cmd=Retrieve&db=PubMed&list_uids=443763&dopt=Abstract

- **Clinical and electroencephalographic study of infantile spasms.**
  Author(s): Anandam R.
  Source: Indian J Pediatr. 1983 September-October; 50(406): 515-8. No Abstract Available.
  http://www.ncbi.nlm.nih.gov:80/entrez/query.fcgi?cmd=Retrieve&db=PubMed&list_uids=6674203&dopt=Abstract

- **Clinical imitators of infantile spasms.**
  Author(s): Donat JF, Wright FS.
  Source: Journal of Child Neurology. 1992 October; 7(4): 395-9.
  http://www.ncbi.nlm.nih.gov:80/entrez/query.fcgi?cmd=Retrieve&db=PubMed&list_uids=1469248&dopt=Abstract

- **Cognitive deficits after cryptogenic infantile spasms with benign seizure evolution.**
  Author(s): Gaily E, Appelqvist K, Kantola-Sorsa E, Liukkonen E, Kyyronen P, Sarpola M, Huttunen H, Valanne L, Granstrom ML.
  Source: Developmental Medicine and Child Neurology. 1999 October; 41(10): 660-4.
  http://www.ncbi.nlm.nih.gov:80/entrez/query.fcgi?cmd=Retrieve&db=PubMed&list_uids=10587041&dopt=Abstract

- **Combination therapy of infantile spasms with high-dose pyridoxal phosphate and low-dose corticotropin.**
  Author(s): Takuma Y, Seki T.
  Source: Journal of Child Neurology. 1996 January; 11(1): 35-40.
  http://www.ncbi.nlm.nih.gov:80/entrez/query.fcgi?cmd=Retrieve&db= PubMed&list_uids=8745383&dopt=Abstract

- **Computed tomography in infantile spasms: effects of hormonal therapy.**
  Author(s): Glaze DG, Hrachovy RA, Frost JD Jr, Zion TE, Bryan RN.
  Source: Pediatric Neurology. 1986 January-February; 2(1): 23-7.
  http://www.ncbi.nlm.nih.gov:80/entrez/query.fcgi?cmd=Retrieve&db= PubMed&list_uids=2854738&dopt=Abstract

- **Computed tomography of infantile spasms.**
  Author(s): Zhang TL, Shao SF, Sha LJ, Zhang T.
  Source: Proc Chin Acad Med Sci Peking Union Med Coll. 1989; 4(3): 172-4. No Abstract Available.
  http://www.ncbi.nlm.nih.gov:80/entrez/query.fcgi?cmd=Retrieve&db= PubMed&list_uids=2594741&dopt=Abstract

- **Computerized tomography of brain in infantile spasms (West syndrome).**
  Author(s): Mahdi AH, Yohannan MD, Patel PJ, Malabarey TM, Kolawole TM.
  Source: Pediatric Radiology. 1990; 21(1): 9-11.
  http://www.ncbi.nlm.nih.gov:80/entrez/query.fcgi?cmd=Retrieve&db= PubMed&list_uids=2287551&dopt=Abstract

- **Confirmation of linkage in X-linked infantile spasms (West syndrome) and refinement of the disease locus to Xp21.3-Xp22.1.**
  Author(s): Bruyere H, Lewis S, Wood S, MacLeod PJ, Langlois S.
  Source: Clinical Genetics. 1999 March; 55(3): 173-81.
  http://www.ncbi.nlm.nih.gov:80/entrez/query.fcgi?cmd=Retrieve&db= PubMed&list_uids=10334471&dopt=Abstract

- **Congenital microcephaly, infantile spasms, psychomotor retardation, and nephrotic syndrome in two sibs.**
  Author(s): Roos RA, Maaswinkel-Mooy PD, vd Loo EM, Kanhai HH.
  Source: European Journal of Pediatrics. 1987 September; 146(5): 532-6.
  http://www.ncbi.nlm.nih.gov:80/entrez/query.fcgi?cmd=Retrieve&db= PubMed&list_uids=3678281&dopt=Abstract

- **Congenital retarded myelinization in a new-born child with infantile spasms.**
  Author(s): de Weerdt CJ, Hooghwinkel GJ.
  Source: Clinical Neurology and Neurosurgery. 1976; 79(2): 143-50.
  http://www.ncbi.nlm.nih.gov:80/entrez/query.fcgi?cmd=Retrieve&db=PubMed&list_uids=1036285&dopt=Abstract

- **Continuous infantile spasms as a form of status epilepticus.**
  Author(s): Coulter DL.
  Source: Journal of Child Neurology. 1986 July; 1(3): 215-7.
  http://www.ncbi.nlm.nih.gov:80/entrez/query.fcgi?cmd=Retrieve&db=PubMed&list_uids=3036934&dopt=Abstract

- **Correction to infantile spasms and Lennox-Gastaut syndrome.**
  Author(s): Trevathan E.
  Source: Journal of Child Neurology. 2003 May; 18(5): 374; Author Reply 374.
  http://www.ncbi.nlm.nih.gov:80/entrez/query.fcgi?cmd=Retrieve&db=PubMed&list_uids=12822828&dopt=Abstract

- **Cortical visual impairment in children with infantile spasms.**
  Author(s): Castano G, Lyons CJ, Jan JE, Connolly M.
  Source: J Aapos. 2000 June; 4(3): 175-8.
  http://www.ncbi.nlm.nih.gov:80/entrez/query.fcgi?cmd=Retrieve&db=PubMed&list_uids=10849395&dopt=Abstract

- **Coupling of focal electrical seizure discharges with infantile spasms: incidence during long-term monitoring in newly diagnosed patients.**
  Author(s): Hrachovy RA, Frost JD Jr, Glaze DG.
  Source: Journal of Clinical Neurophysiology : Official Publication of the American Electroencephalographic Society. 1994 July; 11(4): 461-4.
  http://www.ncbi.nlm.nih.gov:80/entrez/query.fcgi?cmd=Retrieve&db=PubMed&list_uids=7962492&dopt=Abstract

- **Cranial computed tomography in infantile spasms. Primary findings related to long-term mental prognosis.**
  Author(s): Howitz P, Neergaard K, Pedersen H.
  Source: Acta Paediatr Scand. 1990 November; 79(11): 1087-91.
  http://www.ncbi.nlm.nih.gov:80/entrez/query.fcgi?cmd=Retrieve&db=PubMed&list_uids=2176430&dopt=Abstract

- **Critical evaluation of the role of immunization as an etiological factor of infantile spasms.**
  Author(s): Fukuyama Y, Tomori N, Sugitate M.
  Source: Neuropadiatrie. 1977 August; 8(3): 224-37.
  http://www.ncbi.nlm.nih.gov:80/entrez/query.fcgi?cmd=Retrieve&db=PubMed&list_uids=578294&dopt=Abstract

- **CSF protein profile in infantile spasms. Influence of etiology and ACTH or dexamethasone treatment.**
  Author(s): Siemes H, Siegert M, Aksu F, Emrich R, Hanefeld F, Scheffner D.
  Source: Epilepsia. 1984 June; 25(3): 368-76.
  http://www.ncbi.nlm.nih.gov:80/entrez/query.fcgi?cmd=Retrieve&db=PubMed&list_uids=6327252&dopt=Abstract

- **CT and ACTH treatment in infantile spasms.**
  Author(s): Carollo C, Marin G, Scanarini M, Ori C, Drigo P, Casara GL, Laverda AM.
  Source: Childs Brain. 1982 September-October; 9(5): 347-53.
  http://www.ncbi.nlm.nih.gov:80/entrez/query.fcgi?cmd=Retrieve&db=PubMed&list_uids=6290148&dopt=Abstract

- **CT findings of infantile spasms.**
  Author(s): Shinomiya N, Aoki T.
  Source: Folia Psychiatr Neurol Jpn. 1978; 32(3): 393-4. No Abstract Available.
  http://www.ncbi.nlm.nih.gov:80/entrez/query.fcgi?cmd=Retrieve&db=PubMed&list_uids=748124&dopt=Abstract

- **Cushing's ulcer as a consequence of adrenocorticotropic hormone administration for infantile spasms.**
  Author(s): Glauser TA, Rogers M.
  Source: Journal of Child Neurology. 1990 April; 5(2): 111-3.
  http://www.ncbi.nlm.nih.gov:80/entrez/query.fcgi?cmd=Retrieve&db=PubMed&list_uids=2161029&dopt=Abstract

- **Cytomegalovirus infection and infantile spasms.**
  Author(s): Riikonen R.
  Source: Developmental Medicine and Child Neurology. 1978 October; 20(5): 570-9.
  http://www.ncbi.nlm.nih.gov:80/entrez/query.fcgi?cmd=Retrieve&db=PubMed&list_uids=215477&dopt=Abstract

- **Cytomegalovirus infection and infantile spasms.**
  Author(s): Stern H, Latham SC, Tizard JP.
  Source: Lancet. 1968 February 17; 1(7538): 361-2.
  http://www.ncbi.nlm.nih.gov:80/entrez/query.fcgi?cmd=Retrieve&db=PubMed&list_uids=4170186&dopt=Abstract

- **De novo reciprocal translocation t(6;14)(q27;q13.3) in a child with infantile spasms.**
  Author(s): Hattori H, Hayashi K, Okuno T, Temma S, Fujii T, Ochi J, Mikawa H.
  Source: Epilepsia. 1985 July-August; 26(4): 310-3.
  http://www.ncbi.nlm.nih.gov:80/entrez/query.fcgi?cmd=Retrieve&db=PubMed&list_uids=4006889&dopt=Abstract

- **Decrease of N-acetylaspartate after ACTH therapy in patients with infantile spasms.**
  Author(s): Maeda H, Furune S, Nomura K, Kitou O, Ando Y, Negoro T, Watanabe K.
  Source: Neuropediatrics. 1997 October; 28(5): 262-7.
  http://www.ncbi.nlm.nih.gov:80/entrez/query.fcgi?cmd=Retrieve&db=PubMed&list_uids=9413005&dopt=Abstract

- **Decreased cerebrospinal fluid levels of beta-endorphin and ACTH in children with infantile spasms.**
  Author(s): Nagamitsu S, Matsuishi T, Yamashita Y, Shimizu T, Iwanaga R, Murakami Y, Miyazaki M, Hashimoto T, Kato H.
  Source: Journal of Neural Transmission (Vienna, Austria : 1996). 2001; 108(3): 363-71.
  http://www.ncbi.nlm.nih.gov:80/entrez/query.fcgi?cmd=Retrieve&db=PubMed&list_uids=11341487&dopt=Abstract

- **Decreased frequency of seizures in infantile spasms associated with lissencephaly by human herpes virus 7 infection.**
  Author(s): Ono J, Imai K, Tanaka-Taya K, Kurahashi H, Okada S.
  Source: Pediatrics International : Official Journal of the Japan Pediatric Society. 2002 April; 44(2): 168-70.
  http://www.ncbi.nlm.nih.gov:80/entrez/query.fcgi?cmd=Retrieve&db=PubMed&list_uids=11896876&dopt=Abstract

- **Demonstration of four patients with good recovery from infantile spasms and hypsarrhythmia.**
  Author(s): Brandt S, Brammer B.
  Source: Acta Paediatr Scand. 1971 November; 60(6): 729-30. No Abstract Available.
  http://www.ncbi.nlm.nih.gov:80/entrez/query.fcgi?cmd=Retrieve&db=PubMed&list_uids=5123509&dopt=Abstract

- **Dendritic development in neocortex of children with mental defect and infantile spasms.**
  Author(s): Huttenlocher PR.
  Source: Neurology. 1974 March; 24(3): 203-10.
  http://www.ncbi.nlm.nih.gov:80/entrez/query.fcgi?cmd=Retrieve&db=PubMed&list_uids=4130661&dopt=Abstract

- **Developmental outcomes in children receiving resection surgery for medically intractable infantile spasms.**
  Author(s): Asarnow RF, LoPresti C, Guthrie D, Elliott T, Cynn V, Shields WD, Shewmon DA, Sankar R, Peacock WJ.
  Source: Developmental Medicine and Child Neurology. 1997 July; 39(7): 430-40.
  http://www.ncbi.nlm.nih.gov:80/entrez/query.fcgi?cmd=Retrieve&db=PubMed&list_uids=9285433&dopt=Abstract

- **Discharge planning for the child with infantile spasms.**
  Author(s): Kongelbeck SR.
  Source: The Journal of Neuroscience Nursing : Journal of the American Association of Neuroscience Nurses. 1990 August; 22(4): 238-44.
  http://www.ncbi.nlm.nih.gov:80/entrez/query.fcgi?cmd=Retrieve&db=PubMed&list_uids=1697884&dopt=Abstract

- **Disruption of the serine/threonine kinase 9 gene causes severe X-linked infantile spasms and mental retardation.**
  Author(s): Kalscheuer VM, Tao J, Donnelly A, Hollway G, Schwinger E, Kubart S, Menzel C, Hoeltzenbein M, Tommerup N, Eyre H, Harbord M, Haan E, Sutherland GR, Ropers HH, Gecz J.
  Source: American Journal of Human Genetics. 2003 June; 72(6): 1401-11. Epub 2003 May 07.
  http://www.ncbi.nlm.nih.gov:80/entrez/query.fcgi?cmd=Retrieve&db=PubMed&list_uids=12736870&dopt=Abstract

- **Disturbed calcium and phosphate homeostasis during treatment with ACTH of infantile spasms.**
  Author(s): Riikonen R, Simell O, Jaaskelainen J, Rapola J, Perheentupa J.
  Source: Archives of Disease in Childhood. 1986 July; 61(7): 671-6.
  http://www.ncbi.nlm.nih.gov:80/entrez/query.fcgi?cmd=Retrieve&db=PubMed&list_uids=3017235&dopt=Abstract

- **Double-blind study of ACTH vs prednisone therapy in infantile spasms.**
  Author(s): Hrachovy RA, Frost JD Jr, Kellaway P, Zion TE.
  Source: The Journal of Pediatrics. 1983 October; 103(4): 641-5.
  http://www.ncbi.nlm.nih.gov:80/entrez/query.fcgi?cmd=Retrieve&db=PubMed&list_uids=6312008&dopt=Abstract

- **Early clinical and EEG features of infantile spasms in Down syndrome.**
  Author(s): Silva ML, Cieuta C, Guerrini R, Plouin P, Livet MO, Dulac O.
  Source: Epilepsia. 1996 October; 37(10): 977-82.
  http://www.ncbi.nlm.nih.gov:80/entrez/query.fcgi?cmd=Retrieve&db=PubMed&list_uids=8822696&dopt=Abstract

- **Early treatment of infantile spasms (West syndrome) and of myoclonic encephalopathy.**
  Author(s): Gordon N.
  Source: Developmental Medicine and Child Neurology. 1990 April; 32(4): 363.
  http://www.ncbi.nlm.nih.gov:80/entrez/query.fcgi?cmd=Retrieve&db=PubMed&list_uids=2158918&dopt=Abstract

- **Effects of ACTH on brain midline structures in infants with infantile spasms.**
  Author(s): Konishi Y, Hayakawa K, Kuriyama M, Saito M, Fujii Y, Sudo M.
  Source: Pediatric Neurology. 1995 September; 13(2): 134-6.
  http://www.ncbi.nlm.nih.gov:80/entrez/query.fcgi?cmd=Retrieve&db=PubMed&list_uids=8534277&dopt=Abstract

- **Efficacy of the ketogenic diet for infantile spasms.**
  Author(s): Kossoff EH, Pyzik PL, McGrogan JR, Vining EP, Freeman JM.
  Source: Pediatrics. 2002 May; 109(5): 780-3.
  http://www.ncbi.nlm.nih.gov:80/entrez/query.fcgi?cmd=Retrieve&db=PubMed&list_uids=11986436&dopt=Abstract

- **Elevated homovanillic acid in cerebrospinal fluid of children with infantile spasms.**
  Author(s): Ito M, Okuno T, Mikawa H, Osumi Y.
  Source: Epilepsia. 1980 August; 21(4): 387-92.
  http://www.ncbi.nlm.nih.gov:80/entrez/query.fcgi?cmd=Retrieve&db=PubMed&list_uids=6156822&dopt=Abstract

- **Elevated intraocular pressure associated with steroid treatment for infantile spasms.**
  Author(s): Friling R, Weinberger D, Zeharia A, Lusky M, Mimouni M, Gaaton D, Snir M.
  Source: Ophthalmology. 2003 April; 110(4): 831-4.
  http://www.ncbi.nlm.nih.gov:80/entrez/query.fcgi?cmd=Retrieve&db=PubMed&list_uids=12689911&dopt=Abstract

- **Epidemiologic features of infantile spasms in Iceland.**
  Author(s): Luthvigsson P, Olafsson E, Sigurthardottir S, Hauser WA.
  Source: Epilepsia. 1994 July-August; 35(4): 802-5.
  http://www.ncbi.nlm.nih.gov:80/entrez/query.fcgi?cmd=Retrieve&db=PubMed&list_uids=8082625&dopt=Abstract

- **Epidemiologic features of infantile spasms in Slovenia.**
  Author(s): Primec ZR, Kopac S, Neubauer D.
  Source: Epilepsia. 2002 February; 43(2): 183-7.
  http://www.ncbi.nlm.nih.gov:80/entrez/query.fcgi?cmd=Retrieve&db=PubMed&list_uids=11903466&dopt=Abstract

- **Epidemiology of infantile spasms in Sweden.**
  Author(s): Sidenvall R, Eeg-Olofsson O.
  Source: Epilepsia. 1995 June; 36(6): 572-4.
  http://www.ncbi.nlm.nih.gov:80/entrez/query.fcgi?cmd=Retrieve&db=PubMed&list_uids=7555969&dopt=Abstract

- **Epstein-Barr virus infection as a cause of infantile spasms.**
  Author(s): Bialek R, Haverkamp FA, Fichsel H.
  Source: Lancet. 1990 February 17; 335(8686): 425.
  http://www.ncbi.nlm.nih.gov:80/entrez/query.fcgi?cmd=Retrieve&db=PubMed&list_uids=1968164&dopt=Abstract

- **Etiologic classification of infantile spasms in 140 cases: role of positron emission tomography.**
  Author(s): Chugani HT, Conti JR.
  Source: Journal of Child Neurology. 1996 January; 11(1): 44-8.
  http://www.ncbi.nlm.nih.gov:80/entrez/query.fcgi?cmd=Retrieve&db=PubMed&list_uids=8745385&dopt=Abstract

- **Etiology and treatment of infantile spasms: current concepts, including the role of DPT immunization.**
  Author(s): Millichap JG.
  Source: Acta Paediatr Jpn. 1987 February; 29(1): 54-60. No Abstract Available.
  http://www.ncbi.nlm.nih.gov:80/entrez/query.fcgi?cmd=Retrieve&db=PubMed&list_uids=2849852&dopt=Abstract

- **Evidence of late-onset infantile spasms.**
  Author(s): Bednarek N, Motte J, Soufflet C, Plouin P, Dulac O.
  Source: Epilepsia. 1998 January; 39(1): 55-60.
  http://www.ncbi.nlm.nih.gov:80/entrez/query.fcgi?cmd=Retrieve&db=PubMed&list_uids=9578013&dopt=Abstract

- **Evoked potentials in infantile spasms.**
  Author(s): Wenzel D.
  Source: Brain & Development. 1987; 9(4): 365-8.
  http://www.ncbi.nlm.nih.gov:80/entrez/query.fcgi?cmd=Retrieve&db=PubMed&list_uids=3434711&dopt=Abstract

- **Excitatory amino acid levels in cerebrospinal fluid of patients with infantile spasms.**
  Author(s): Ince E, Karagol U, Deda G.
  Source: Acta Paediatrica (Oslo, Norway : 1992). 1997 December; 86(12): 1333-6.
  http://www.ncbi.nlm.nih.gov:80/entrez/query.fcgi?cmd=Retrieve&db=PubMed&list_uids=9475311&dopt=Abstract

- **Facilitation of infantile spasms by partial seizures.**
  Author(s): Carrazana EJ, Lombroso CT, Mikati M, Helmers S, Holmes GL.
  Source: Epilepsia. 1993 January-February; 34(1): 97-109.
  http://www.ncbi.nlm.nih.gov:80/entrez/query.fcgi?cmd=Retrieve&db=PubMed&list_uids=8422869&dopt=Abstract

- **Fatal Pneumocystis pneumonia from ACTH therapy for infantile spasms.**
  Author(s): Goetting MG.
  Source: Annals of Neurology. 1986 March; 19(3): 307-8.
  http://www.ncbi.nlm.nih.gov:80/entrez/query.fcgi?cmd=Retrieve&db=PubMed&list_uids=3008640&dopt=Abstract

- **Felbamate for refractory infantile spasms.**
  Author(s): Hosain S, Nagarajan L, Carson D, Solomon G, Mast J, Labar D.
  Source: Journal of Child Neurology. 1997 October; 12(7): 466-8.
  http://www.ncbi.nlm.nih.gov:80/entrez/query.fcgi?cmd=Retrieve&db=PubMed&list_uids=9373806&dopt=Abstract

- **Fibromatosis of dura presenting as infantile spasms.**
  Author(s): Dolman CL, Crichton JU, Jones EA, Lapointe J.
  Source: Journal of the Neurological Sciences. 1981 January; 49(1): 31-9.
  http://www.ncbi.nlm.nih.gov:80/entrez/query.fcgi?cmd=Retrieve&db=PubMed&list_uids=7205317&dopt=Abstract

- **Findings of computed tomography in cases of infantile spasms and Lennox syndrome.**
  Author(s): Imamura S, Sogawa H.
  Source: Folia Psychiatr Neurol Jpn. 1980; 34(3): 385. No Abstract Available.
  http://www.ncbi.nlm.nih.gov:80/entrez/query.fcgi?cmd=Retrieve&db=PubMed&list_uids=6783493&dopt=Abstract

- **Focal and global cortical hypometabolism in patients with newly diagnosed infantile spasms.**
  Author(s): Cochrane Database Syst Rev. 2003;(3):CD001770
  Source: Neurology. 2002 June 11; 58(11): 1646-51.
  /entrez/query.fcgi?cmd=Retrieve&db=pubmed&dopt=Abstract&list_uids=12917912

- **Focal segmental glomerulosclerosis associated with infantile spasms in five mentally retarded children: a morphological analysis on mesangiolysis.**
  Author(s): Joh K, Usui N, Aizawa S, Yamaguchi Y, Chiba S, Takahashi T, Muramatsu Y, Sakai S.
  Source: American Journal of Kidney Diseases : the Official Journal of the National Kidney Foundation. 1991 May; 17(5): 569-77.
  http://www.ncbi.nlm.nih.gov:80/entrez/query.fcgi?cmd=Retrieve&db=PubMed&list_uids=2024658&dopt=Abstract

- **Free amino acids in cerebrospinal fluid from patients with infantile spasms.**
  Author(s): Spink DC, Snead OC 3rd, Swann JW, Martin DL.
  Source: Epilepsia. 1988 May-June; 29(3): 300-6.
  http://www.ncbi.nlm.nih.gov:80/entrez/query.fcgi?cmd=Retrieve&db=PubMed&list_uids=2897288&dopt=Abstract

- **Further observations on the treatment of infantile spasms with corticotropin.**
  Author(s): Fois A, Malandrini F, Mostardini R.
  Source: Brain & Development. 1987; 9(2): 82-4.
  http://www.ncbi.nlm.nih.gov:80/entrez/query.fcgi?cmd=Retrieve&db=PubMed&list_uids=2820258&dopt=Abstract

- **Ganaxolone for treating intractable infantile spasms: a multicenter, open-label, add-on trial.**
  Author(s): Kerrigan JF, Shields WD, Nelson TY, Bluestone DL, Dodson WE, Bourgeois BF, Pellock JM, Morton LD, Monaghan EP.
  Source: Epilepsy Research. 2000 December; 42(2-3): 133-9.
  http://www.ncbi.nlm.nih.gov:80/entrez/query.fcgi?cmd=Retrieve&db=PubMed&list_uids=11074186&dopt=Abstract

- **Gene expression analysis as a strategy to understand the molecular pathogenesis of infantile spasms.**
  Author(s): Crino PB.
  Source: Int Rev Neurobiol. 2002; 49: 367-89. Review. No Abstract Available.
  http://www.ncbi.nlm.nih.gov:80/entrez/query.fcgi?cmd=Retrieve&db=PubMed&list_uids=12040902&dopt=Abstract

- **Generators of ictal and interictal electroencephalograms associated with infantile spasms: intracellular studies of cortical and thalamic neurons.**
  Author(s): Steriade M, Timofeev I.
  Source: Int Rev Neurobiol. 2002; 49: 77-98. Review. No Abstract Available.
  http://www.ncbi.nlm.nih.gov:80/entrez/query.fcgi?cmd=Retrieve&db=PubMed&list_uids=12040907&dopt=Abstract

- **High dose B6 treatment in infantile spasms.**
  Author(s): Blennow G, Starck L.
  Source: Neuropediatrics. 1986 February; 17(1): 7-10.
  http://www.ncbi.nlm.nih.gov:80/entrez/query.fcgi?cmd=Retrieve&db=PubMed&list_uids=3960285&dopt=Abstract

- **High-dose corticotropin (ACTH) versus prednisone for infantile spasms: a prospective, randomized, blinded study.**
  Author(s): Baram TZ, Mitchell WG, Tournay A, Snead OC, Hanson RA, Horton EJ.
  Source: Pediatrics. 1996 March; 97(3): 375-9.
  http://www.ncbi.nlm.nih.gov:80/entrez/query.fcgi?cmd=Retrieve&db=PubMed&list_uids=8604274&dopt=Abstract

- **High-dose, long-duration versus low-dose, short-duration corticotropin therapy for infantile spasms.**
  Author(s): Hrachovy RA, Frost JD Jr, Glaze DG.
  Source: The Journal of Pediatrics. 1994 May; 124(5 Pt 1): 803-6.
  http://www.ncbi.nlm.nih.gov:80/entrez/query.fcgi?cmd=Retrieve&db=PubMed&list_uids=8176573&dopt=Abstract

- **Histopathology of brain tissue from patients with infantile spasms.**
  Author(s): Vinters HV.
  Source: Int Rev Neurobiol. 2002; 49: 63-76. Review.
  http://www.ncbi.nlm.nih.gov:80/entrez/query.fcgi?cmd=Retrieve&db=PubMed&list_uids=12040906&dopt=Abstract

- **Home care management of the child with infantile spasms.**
  Author(s): Kolodgie MJ.
  Source: Pediatric Nursing. 1994 May-June; 20(3): 270-3, 259.
  http://www.ncbi.nlm.nih.gov:80/entrez/query.fcgi?cmd=Retrieve&db=PubMed&list_uids=8008476&dopt=Abstract

- **Homocarnosine levels in cerebrospinal fluid of patients with infantile spasms under ACTH therapy.**
  Author(s): Ohtsuka C, Sato Y, Takahashi H.
  Source: Brain & Development. 1983; 5(5): 464-8.
  http://www.ncbi.nlm.nih.gov:80/entrez/query.fcgi?cmd=Retrieve&db=PubMed&list_uids=6318586&dopt=Abstract

- **How do cryptogenic and symptomatic infantile spasms differ? Review of biochemical studies in Finnish patients.**
  Author(s): Riikonen RS.
  Source: Journal of Child Neurology. 1996 September; 11(5): 383-8.
  http://www.ncbi.nlm.nih.gov:80/entrez/query.fcgi?cmd=Retrieve&db=PubMed&list_uids=8877606&dopt=Abstract

- **How does ACTH work against infantile spasms? Bedside to bench.**
  Author(s): Snead OC 3rd.
  Source: Annals of Neurology. 2001 March; 49(3): 288-9.
  http://www.ncbi.nlm.nih.gov:80/entrez/query.fcgi?cmd=Retrieve&db=PubMed&list_uids=11261501&dopt=Abstract

- **Human herpesvirus-6 associated encephalitis with subsequent infantile spasms and cerebellar astrocytoma.**
  Author(s): Rantala H, Mannonen L, Ahtiluoto S, Linnavuori K, Herva R, Vaheri A, Koskiniemi M.
  Source: Developmental Medicine and Child Neurology. 2000 June; 42(6): 418-21.
  http://www.ncbi.nlm.nih.gov:80/entrez/query.fcgi?cmd=Retrieve&db=PubMed&list_uids=10875530&dopt=Abstract

- **Hyperkalemia as a late side effect of prolonged adrenocorticotropic hormone therapy for infantile spasms.**
  Author(s): Zeharia A, Levy Y, Rachmel A, Nitzan M, Steinherz R.
  Source: Helv Paediatr Acta. 1987 June; 42(5-6): 433-6.
  http://www.ncbi.nlm.nih.gov:80/entrez/query.fcgi?cmd=Retrieve&db=PubMed&list_uids=3136101&dopt=Abstract

- **Hypertrophic cardiomyopathy during corticotropin therapy for infantile spasms. A clinical and echocardiographic study.**
  Author(s): Bobele GB, Ward KE, Bodensteiner JB.
  Source: Am J Dis Child. 1993 February; 147(2): 223-5.
  http://www.ncbi.nlm.nih.gov:80/entrez/query.fcgi?cmd=Retrieve&db=PubMed&list_uids=8381257&dopt=Abstract

- **Hypothalamo-pituitary-adrenal function in infantile spasms: effects of ACTH therapy.**
  Author(s): Rao JK, Willis J.
  Source: Journal of Child Neurology. 1987 July; 2(3): 220-3.
  http://www.ncbi.nlm.nih.gov:80/entrez/query.fcgi?cmd=Retrieve&db=PubMed&list_uids=3038989&dopt=Abstract

- **Hypotony in children with infantile spasms.**
  Author(s): Holub V, Zakova E, Zemanova H.
  Source: Acta Univ Carol Med Monogr. 1976; (75): 45-6. No Abstract Available.
  http://www.ncbi.nlm.nih.gov:80/entrez/query.fcgi?cmd=Retrieve&db=PubMed&list_uids=1052642&dopt=Abstract

- **Hypsarhythmia-infantile spasms in near-drowning: clinical, EEG, CT scan and evoked potential studies.**
  Author(s): Ganji S, Tilton AC, Happel L, Marino S.
  Source: Clin Electroencephalogr. 1987 October; 18(4): 180-6.
  http://www.ncbi.nlm.nih.gov:80/entrez/query.fcgi?cmd=Retrieve&db=PubMed&list_uids=3665108&dopt=Abstract

- **Hysarhythmia: infantile spasms.**
  Author(s): Robins MH.
  Source: J Am Osteopath Assoc. 1968 April; 67(8): 882-8. No Abstract Available.
  http://www.ncbi.nlm.nih.gov:80/entrez/query.fcgi?cmd=Retrieve&db=PubMed&list_uids=5185264&dopt=Abstract

- **Ictal pattern of EEG and muscular activation in symptomatic infantile spasms: a videopolygraphic and computer analysis.**
  Author(s): Bisulli F, Volpi L, Meletti S, Rubboli G, Franzoni E, Moscano M, d'Orsi G, Tassinari CA.
  Source: Epilepsia. 2002 December; 43(12): 1559-63.
  http://www.ncbi.nlm.nih.gov:80/entrez/query.fcgi?cmd=Retrieve&db=PubMed&list_uids=12460259&dopt=Abstract

- **Immunohistochemical analysis of brainstem lesions in infantile spasms.**
  Author(s): Hayashi M, Itoh M, Araki S, Kumada S, Tanuma N, Kohji T, Kohyama J, Iwakawa Y, Satoh J, Morimatsu Y.
  Source: Neuropathology : Official Journal of the Japanese Society of Neuropathology. 2000 December; 20(4): 297-303.
  http://www.ncbi.nlm.nih.gov:80/entrez/query.fcgi?cmd=Retrieve&db=PubMed&list_uids=11211054&dopt=Abstract

- **Infantile spasms and Lennox-Gastaut syndrome.**
  Author(s): Trevathan E.
  Source: Journal of Child Neurology. 2002 February; 17 Suppl 2: 2S9-2S22. Review. Erratum In: J Child Neurol. 2003 May; 18(5): 374.
  http://www.ncbi.nlm.nih.gov:80/entrez/query.fcgi?cmd=Retrieve&db=PubMed&list_uids=11952036&dopt=Abstract

- **Infantile spasms and Menkes disease.**
  Author(s): Sfaello I, Castelnau P, Blanc N, Ogier H, Evrard P, Arzimanoglou A.
  Source: Epileptic Disorders : International Epilepsy Journal with Videotape. 2000 December; 2(4): 227-30.
  http://www.ncbi.nlm.nih.gov:80/entrez/query.fcgi?cmd=Retrieve&db=PubMed&list_uids=11174154&dopt=Abstract

- **Infantile spasms and vigabatrin. Study will compare effects of drugs.**
  Author(s): Osborne JP, Edwards SW, Hancock E, Lux AL, O'Callaghan F, Johnson T, Kennedy CR, Newton RW, Verity CM.
  Source: Bmj (Clinical Research Ed.). 1999 January 2; 318(7175): 56-7.
  http://www.ncbi.nlm.nih.gov:80/entrez/query.fcgi?cmd=Retrieve&db=PubMed&list_uids=9872899&dopt=Abstract

- **Infantile spasms and vigabatrin. Visual field defects may be permanent.**
  Author(s): Lhatoo SD, Sander JW.
  Source: Bmj (Clinical Research Ed.). 1999 January 2; 318(7175): 57.
  http://www.ncbi.nlm.nih.gov:80/entrez/query.fcgi?cmd=Retrieve&db=PubMed&list_uids=10068225&dopt=Abstract

- **Infantile spasms as a cause of acquired perinatal visual loss.**
  Author(s): Brooks BP, Simpson JL, Leber SM, Robertson PL, Archer SM.
  Source: J Aapos. 2002 December; 6(6): 385-8.
  http://www.ncbi.nlm.nih.gov:80/entrez/query.fcgi?cmd=Retrieve&db=PubMed&list_uids=12506281&dopt=Abstract

- **Infantile spasms associated with a histamine H1 antagonist.**
  Author(s): Yasuhara A, Ochi A, Harada Y, Kobayashi Y.
  Source: Neuropediatrics. 1998 December; 29(6): 320-1.
  http://www.ncbi.nlm.nih.gov:80/entrez/query.fcgi?cmd=Retrieve&db=PubMed&list_uids=10029352&dopt=Abstract

- **Infantile spasms in a patient with partial duplication of chromosome 2p.**
  Author(s): Kubo T, Kakinuma H, Nakamura T, Kitatani M, Ozaki M, Takahashi H.
  Source: Clinical Genetics. 1999 July; 56(1): 93-4.
  http://www.ncbi.nlm.nih.gov:80/entrez/query.fcgi?cmd=Retrieve&db=PubMed&list_uids=10466424&dopt=Abstract

- **Infantile spasms in a patient with williams syndrome and craniosynostosis.**
  Author(s): Morimoto M, An B, Ogami A, Shin N, Sugino Y, Sawai Y, Usuku T, Tanaka M, Hirai K, Nishimura A, Hasegawa K, Sugimoto T.
  Source: Epilepsia. 2003 November; 44(11): 1459-62.
  http://www.ncbi.nlm.nih.gov:80/entrez/query.fcgi?cmd=Retrieve&db=PubMed&list_uids=14636357&dopt=Abstract

- **Infantile spasms in Down syndrome: good response to a short course of vigabatrin.**
  Author(s): Nabbout R, Melki I, Gerbaka B, Dulac O, Akatcherian C.
  Source: Epilepsia. 2001 December; 42(12): 1580-3.
  http://www.ncbi.nlm.nih.gov:80/entrez/query.fcgi?cmd=Retrieve&db=PubMed&list_uids=11879370&dopt=Abstract

- **Infantile spasms in Down syndrome--effects of delayed anticonvulsive treatment.**
  Author(s): Eisermann MM, DeLaRaillere A, Dellatolas G, Tozzi E, Nabbout R, Dulac O, Chiron C.
  Source: Epilepsy Research. 2003 June-July; 55(1-2): 21-7.
  http://www.ncbi.nlm.nih.gov:80/entrez/query.fcgi?cmd=Retrieve&db=PubMed&list_uids=12948613&dopt=Abstract

- **Infantile spasms in remission may reemerge as intractable epileptic spasms.**
  Author(s): Camfield P, Camfield C, Lortie A, Darwish H.
  Source: Epilepsia. 2003 December; 44(12): 1592-5.
  http://www.ncbi.nlm.nih.gov:80/entrez/query.fcgi?cmd=Retrieve&db=PubMed&list_uids=14636334&dopt=Abstract

- **Infantile spasms in tuberous sclerosis complex.**
  Author(s): Curatolo P, Seri S, Verdecchia M, Bombardieri R.
  Source: Brain & Development. 2001 November; 23(7): 502-7. Review.
  http://www.ncbi.nlm.nih.gov:80/entrez/query.fcgi?cmd=Retrieve&db=PubMed&list_uids=11701245&dopt=Abstract

- **Infantile spasms versus myoclonus: is there a connection?**
  Author(s): Pranzatelli MR.
  Source: Int Rev Neurobiol. 2002; 49: 285-314. Review.
  http://www.ncbi.nlm.nih.gov:80/entrez/query.fcgi?cmd=Retrieve&db=PubMed&list_uids=12040898&dopt=Abstract

- **Infantile spasms with basal ganglia MRI hypersignal may reveal mitochondrial disorder due to T8993G MT DNA mutation.**
  Author(s): Desguerre I, Pinton F, Nabbout R, Moutard ML, N'Guyen S, Marsac C, Ponsot G, Dulac O.
  Source: Neuropediatrics. 2003 June; 34(5): 265-9.
  http://www.ncbi.nlm.nih.gov:80/entrez/query.fcgi?cmd=Retrieve&db=PubMed&list_uids=14598233&dopt=Abstract

- **Infantile spasms, dystonia, and other X-linked phenotypes caused by mutations in Aristaless related homeobox gene, ARX.**
  Author(s): Stromme P, Mangelsdorf ME, Scheffer IE, Gecz J.
  Source: Brain & Development. 2002 August; 24(5): 266-8.
  http://www.ncbi.nlm.nih.gov:80/entrez/query.fcgi?cmd=Retrieve&db=PubMed&list_uids=12142061&dopt=Abstract

- **Infantile spasms.**
  Author(s): Zupanc ML.
  Source: Expert Opinion on Pharmacotherapy. 2003 November; 4(11): 2039-48. Review.
  http://www.ncbi.nlm.nih.gov:80/entrez/query.fcgi?cmd=Retrieve&db=PubMed&list_uids=14596657&dopt=Abstract

- **Infantile spasms.**
  Author(s): Wong M, Trevathan E.
  Source: Pediatric Neurology. 2001 February; 24(2): 89-98. Review.
  http://www.ncbi.nlm.nih.gov:80/entrez/query.fcgi?cmd=Retrieve&db=PubMed&list_uids=11275456&dopt=Abstract

- **Infantile spasms: a proposal for a staged evaluation.**
  Author(s): Trasmonte JV, Barron TF.
  Source: Pediatric Neurology. 1998 November; 19(5): 368-71.
  http://www.ncbi.nlm.nih.gov:80/entrez/query.fcgi?cmd=Retrieve&db=PubMed&list_uids=9880142&dopt=Abstract

- **Infantile spasms: criteria for an animal model.**
  Author(s): Stafstrom CE, Holmes GL.
  Source: Int Rev Neurobiol. 2002; 49: 391-411. Review.
  http://www.ncbi.nlm.nih.gov:80/entrez/query.fcgi?cmd=Retrieve&db=PubMed&list_uids=12040904&dopt=Abstract

- **Infantile spasms: diagnosis and assessment of treatment response by video-EEG.**
  Author(s): Gaily E, Liukkonen E, Paetau R, Rekola R, Granstrom ML.
  Source: Developmental Medicine and Child Neurology. 2001 October; 43(10): 658-67.
  http://www.ncbi.nlm.nih.gov:80/entrez/query.fcgi?cmd=Retrieve&db=PubMed&list_uids=11665822&dopt=Abstract

- **Infantile spasms: facial expression of affect before and after epilepsy surgery.**
  Author(s): Caplan R, Guthrie D, Komo S, Shields WD, Sigman M.
  Source: Brain and Cognition. 1999 March; 39(2): 116-32.
  http://www.ncbi.nlm.nih.gov:80/entrez/query.fcgi?cmd=Retrieve&db=PubMed&list_uids=10079120&dopt=Abstract

- **Infantile spasms: hypothesis-driven therapy and pilot human infant experiments using corticotropin-releasing hormone receptor antagonists.**
  Author(s): Baram TZ, Mitchell WG, Brunson K, Haden E.
  Source: Developmental Neuroscience. 1999 November; 21(3-5): 281-9.
  http://www.ncbi.nlm.nih.gov:80/entrez/query.fcgi?cmd=Retrieve&db=PubMed&list_uids=10575251&dopt=Abstract

- **Infantile spasms: the development of nonverbal communication after epilepsy surgery.**
  Author(s): Caplan R, Guthrie D, Komo S, Shields WD, Sigmann M.
  Source: Developmental Neuroscience. 1999 November; 21(3-5): 165-73.
  http://www.ncbi.nlm.nih.gov:80/entrez/query.fcgi?cmd=Retrieve&db=PubMed&list_uids=10575239&dopt=Abstract

- **Infantile spasms: the original description of Dr West. 1841.**
  Author(s): Duncan R.
  Source: Epileptic Disorders : International Epilepsy Journal with Videotape. 2001 January-March; 3(1): 47-8.
  http://www.ncbi.nlm.nih.gov:80/entrez/query.fcgi?cmd=Retrieve&db=PubMed&list_uids=11313223&dopt=Abstract

- **Infantile spasms: unique syndrome or general age-dependent manifestation of a diffuse encephalopathy?**
  Author(s): Koehn MA, Duchowny M.
  Source: Int Rev Neurobiol. 2002; 49: 57-62. Review. No Abstract Available.
  http://www.ncbi.nlm.nih.gov:80/entrez/query.fcgi?cmd=Retrieve&db=PubMed&list_uids=12040905&dopt=Abstract

- **Infantile spasms: West syndrome.**
  Author(s): Carmant L.
  Source: Archives of Neurology. 2002 February; 59(2): 317-8.
  http://www.ncbi.nlm.nih.gov:80/entrez/query.fcgi?cmd=Retrieve&db=PubMed&list_uids=11843708&dopt=Abstract

- **Informative value of magnetic resonance imaging and EEG in the prognosis of infantile spasms.**
  Author(s): Saltik S, Kocer N, Dervent A.
  Source: Epilepsia. 2002 March; 43(3): 246-52.
  http://www.ncbi.nlm.nih.gov:80/entrez/query.fcgi?cmd=Retrieve&db=PubMed&list_uids=11906509&dopt=Abstract

- **Interstitial deletion of chromosome 7q in a patient with Williams syndrome and infantile spasms.**
  Author(s): Mizugishi K, Yamanaka K, Kuwajima K, Kondo I.
  Source: Journal of Human Genetics. 1998; 43(3): 178-81.
  http://www.ncbi.nlm.nih.gov:80/entrez/query.fcgi?cmd=Retrieve&db=PubMed&list_uids=9747030&dopt=Abstract

- **Kynurenic acid is decreased in cerebrospinal fluid of patients with infantile spasms.**
  Author(s): Yamamoto H, Shindo I, Egawa B, Horiguchi K.
  Source: Pediatric Neurology. 1994 February; 10(1): 9-12.
  http://www.ncbi.nlm.nih.gov:80/entrez/query.fcgi?cmd=Retrieve&db=PubMed&list_uids=8198681&dopt=Abstract

- **Lack of clinical-EEG effects of naloxone injection on infantile spasms.**
  Author(s): Nalin A, Petraglia F, Genazzani AR, Frigieri G, Facchinetti F.
  Source: Child's Nervous System : Chns : Official Journal of the International Society for Pediatric Neurosurgery. 1988 December; 4(6): 365-6.
  http://www.ncbi.nlm.nih.gov:80/entrez/query.fcgi?cmd=Retrieve&db=PubMed&list_uids=3245947&dopt=Abstract

- **Lactic dehydrogenase isoenzyme in cerebrospinal fluid of children with infantile spasms.**
  Author(s): Nussinovitch M, Harel D, Eidlitz-Markus T, Amir J, Volovitz B.
  Source: European Neurology. 2003; 49(4): 231-3.
  http://www.ncbi.nlm.nih.gov:80/entrez/query.fcgi?cmd=Retrieve&db=PubMed&list_uids=12736540&dopt=Abstract

- **Lamotrigine in infantile spasms.**
  Author(s): Veggiotti P, Cieuta C, Rex E, Dulac O.
  Source: Lancet. 1994 November 12; 344(8933): 1375-6.
  http://www.ncbi.nlm.nih.gov:80/entrez/query.fcgi?cmd=Retrieve&db=PubMed&list_uids=7968065&dopt=Abstract

- **Leigh syndrome, cytochrome C oxidase deficiency and hypsarrhythmia with infantile spasms.**
  Author(s): Tsao CY, Luquette M, Rusin JA, Herr GM, Kien CL, Morrow G 3rd.
  Source: Clin Electroencephalogr. 1997 October; 28(4): 214-7.
  http://www.ncbi.nlm.nih.gov:80/entrez/query.fcgi?cmd=Retrieve&db=PubMed&list_uids=9343714&dopt=Abstract

- **Leigh's subacute necrotizing encephalomyelopathy in a child with infantile spasms and hypsarrhythmia.**
  Author(s): Kamoshita S, Mizutani I, Fukuyama Y.
  Source: Developmental Medicine and Child Neurology. 1970 August; 12(4): 430-5.
  http://www.ncbi.nlm.nih.gov:80/entrez/query.fcgi?cmd=Retrieve&db=PubMed&list_uids=5457538&dopt=Abstract

- **Letter: Infantile spasms and cytomegalovirus infection.**
  Author(s): Midulla M, Balducci L, Iannetti P, Businco L, Rezza E, Fois A.
  Source: Lancet. 1976 August 14; 2(7981): 377.
  http://www.ncbi.nlm.nih.gov:80/entrez/query.fcgi?cmd=Retrieve&db=PubMed&list_uids=60616&dopt=Abstract

- **Letter: Infantile spasms and subsequent appearance of tuberous sclerosis syndrome.**
  Author(s): Pampiglione G, Pugh E.
  Source: Lancet. 1975 November 22; 2(7943): 1046.
  http://www.ncbi.nlm.nih.gov:80/entrez/query.fcgi?cmd=Retrieve&db=PubMed&list_uids=53537&dopt=Abstract

- **Linea nevus sebaceus. A neurocutaneous syndrome associated with infantile spasms.**
  Author(s): Herbst BA, Cohen ME.
  Source: Archives of Neurology. 1971 April; 24(4): 317-22.
  http://www.ncbi.nlm.nih.gov:80/entrez/query.fcgi?cmd=Retrieve&db=PubMed&list_uids=5548451&dopt=Abstract

- **Linear nevus sebaceus syndrome. Report of a case with Lennox-Gastaut syndrome following infantile spasms.**
  Author(s): Kurokawa T, Sasaki K, Hanai T, Goya N, Komaki S.
  Source: Archives of Neurology. 1981 June; 38(6): 375-7.
  http://www.ncbi.nlm.nih.gov:80/entrez/query.fcgi?cmd=Retrieve&db=PubMed&list_uids=6972208&dopt=Abstract

- **Localization of focal cortical lesions influences age of onset of infantile spasms.**
  Author(s): Koo B, Hwang P.
  Source: Epilepsia. 1996 November; 37(11): 1068-71.
  http://www.ncbi.nlm.nih.gov:80/entrez/query.fcgi?cmd=Retrieve&db=PubMed&list_uids=8917056&dopt=Abstract

- **Long term changes in patients with hypsarrhythmia-infantile spasms: 505 patients, up to 43 years follow-up.**
  Author(s): Hughes JR, Rechitsky I, Daaboul Y.
  Source: Clin Electroencephalogr. 1997 January; 28(1): 1-15.
  http://www.ncbi.nlm.nih.gov:80/entrez/query.fcgi?cmd=Retrieve&db=PubMed&list_uids=9013045&dopt=Abstract

- **Long-term otucome of West syndrome: a study of adults with a history of infantile spasms.**
  Author(s): Riikonen R.
  Source: Epilepsia. 1996 April; 37(4): 367-72.
  http://www.ncbi.nlm.nih.gov:80/entrez/query.fcgi?cmd=Retrieve&db=PubMed&list_uids=8603642&dopt=Abstract

- **Long-term outcomes of conventional therapy for infantile spasms.**
  Author(s): Holden KR, Clarke SL, Griesemer DA.
  Source: Seizure : the Journal of the British Epilepsy Association. 1997 June; 6(3): 201-5.
  http://www.ncbi.nlm.nih.gov:80/entrez/query.fcgi?cmd=Retrieve&db=PubMed&list_uids=9203248&dopt=Abstract

- **Long-term prognosis after infantile spasms: a statistical study of prognostic factors in 200 cases.**
  Author(s): Matsumoto A, Watanabe K, Negoro T, Sugiura M, Iwase K, Hara K, Miyazaki S.
  Source: Developmental Medicine and Child Neurology. 1981 February; 23(1): 51-65.
  http://www.ncbi.nlm.nih.gov:80/entrez/query.fcgi?cmd=Retrieve&db=PubMed&list_uids=6259007&dopt=Abstract

- **Long-term prognosis in infantile spasms: a follow-up report on 112 cases.**
  Author(s): Jeavons PM, Harper JR, Bower BD.
  Source: Developmental Medicine and Child Neurology. 1970 August; 12(4): 413-21.
  http://www.ncbi.nlm.nih.gov:80/entrez/query.fcgi?cmd=Retrieve&db=PubMed&list_uids=5457536&dopt=Abstract

- **Long-term prognosis of 200 cases of infantile spasms. Part II: Electroencephalographic findings at the ages between 5-7.**
  Author(s): Negoro T, Matsumoto A, Sugiura M, Iwase K, Watanabe K, Hara K, Miyazaki S.
  Source: Folia Psychiatr Neurol Jpn. 1980; 34(3): 346-7. No Abstract Available.
  http://www.ncbi.nlm.nih.gov:80/entrez/query.fcgi?cmd=Retrieve&db=PubMed&list_uids=7216038&dopt=Abstract

- **Long-term prognosis of patients with infantile spasms following ACTH therapy.**
  Author(s): Pollack MA, Zion TE, Kellaway P.
  Source: Epilepsia. 1979 June; 20(3): 255-60.
  http://www.ncbi.nlm.nih.gov:80/entrez/query.fcgi?cmd=Retrieve&db=PubMed&list_uids=221212&dopt=Abstract

- **Magnetic resonance imaging findings in infantile spasms: etiologic and pathophysiologic aspects.**
  Author(s): Saltik S, Kocer N, Dervent A.
  Source: Journal of Child Neurology. 2003 April; 18(4): 241-6.
  http://www.ncbi.nlm.nih.gov:80/entrez/query.fcgi?cmd=Retrieve&db=PubMed&list_uids=12760425&dopt=Abstract

- **Magnetic resonance imaging in infantile spasms: effects of hormonal therapy.**
  Author(s): Konishi Y, Yasujima M, Kuriyama M, Konishi K, Hayakawa K, Fujii Y, Ishii Y, Sudo M.
  Source: Epilepsia. 1992 March-April; 33(2): 304-9.
  http://www.ncbi.nlm.nih.gov:80/entrez/query.fcgi?cmd=Retrieve&db=PubMed&list_uids=1312459&dopt=Abstract

- **Medical treatment of patients with infantile spasms.**
  Author(s): Mikati MA, Lepejian GA, Holmes GL.
  Source: Clinical Neuropharmacology. 2002 March-April; 25(2): 61-70. Review.
  http://www.ncbi.nlm.nih.gov:80/entrez/query.fcgi?cmd=Retrieve&db=PubMed&list_uids=11981230&dopt=Abstract

- **Microscopic cortical dysplasia in infantile spasms: evolution of white matter abnormalities.**
  Author(s): Sankar R, Curran JG, Kevill JW, Rintahaka PJ, Shewmon DA, Vinters HV.
  Source: Ajnr. American Journal of Neuroradiology. 1995 June-July; 16(6): 1265-72.
  http://www.ncbi.nlm.nih.gov:80/entrez/query.fcgi?cmd=Retrieve&db= PubMed&list_uids=7677022&dopt=Abstract

- **Mitochondrial disorders: a potentially under-recognized etiology of infantile spasms.**
  Author(s): Shah NS, Mitchell WG, Boles RG.
  Source: Journal of Child Neurology. 2002 May; 17(5): 369-72.
  http://www.ncbi.nlm.nih.gov:80/entrez/query.fcgi?cmd=Retrieve&db= PubMed&list_uids=12150585&dopt=Abstract

- **Mogadon therapy of infantile spasms.**
  Author(s): Weinmann HM.
  Source: Electroencephalography and Clinical Neurophysiology. 1967 August; 23(2): 183.
  http://www.ncbi.nlm.nih.gov:80/entrez/query.fcgi?cmd=Retrieve&db= PubMed&list_uids=4166705&dopt=Abstract

- **Morphological aspects of aetiology and the course of infantile spasms (West-syndrome).**
  Author(s): Meencke HJ, Gerhard C.
  Source: Neuropediatrics. 1985 May; 16(2): 59-66.
  http://www.ncbi.nlm.nih.gov:80/entrez/query.fcgi?cmd=Retrieve&db= PubMed&list_uids=3925364&dopt=Abstract

- **Morphological substrates of infantile spasms: studies based on surgically resected cerebral tissue.**
  Author(s): Vinters HV, Fisher RS, Cornford ME, Mah V, Secor DL, De Rosa MJ, Comair YG, Peacock WJ, Shields WD.
  Source: Child's Nervous System : Chns : Official Journal of the International Society for Pediatric Neurosurgery. 1992 February; 8(1): 8-17.
  http://www.ncbi.nlm.nih.gov:80/entrez/query.fcgi?cmd=Retrieve&db= PubMed&list_uids=1315619&dopt=Abstract

- **Myoclonic infantile spasms.**
  Author(s): Russo P, Bakke K.
  Source: The Nurse Practitioner. 1977 September-October; 4(5): 26, 28-30.
  http://www.ncbi.nlm.nih.gov:80/entrez/query.fcgi?cmd=Retrieve&db=
  PubMed&list_uids=226911&dopt=Abstract

- **Neonatal hemangiomatosis presenting as infantile spasms.**
  Author(s): McShane MA, Finn JP, Hall-Craggs MA, Hanmer O, Harper J.
  Source: Neuropediatrics. 1990 November; 21(4): 211-2.
  http://www.ncbi.nlm.nih.gov:80/entrez/query.fcgi?cmd=Retrieve&db=
  PubMed&list_uids=2290483&dopt=Abstract

- **Neuropathologic study of resected cerebral tissue from patients with infantile spasms.**
  Author(s): Vinters HV, De Rosa MJ, Farrell MA.
  Source: Epilepsia. 1993 July-August; 34(4): 772-9.
  http://www.ncbi.nlm.nih.gov:80/entrez/query.fcgi?cmd=Retrieve&db=
  PubMed&list_uids=8330591&dopt=Abstract

- **Neuropathological aspects of infantile spasms.**
  Author(s): Jellinger K.
  Source: Brain & Development. 1987; 9(4): 349-57. Review.
  http://www.ncbi.nlm.nih.gov:80/entrez/query.fcgi?cmd=Retrieve&db=
  PubMed&list_uids=3324792&dopt=Abstract

- **Neuropathology of the brainstem in age-dependent epileptic encephalopathy--especially of cases with infantile spasms.**
  Author(s): Satoh J, Mizutani T, Morimatsu Y.
  Source: Brain & Development. 1986; 8(4): 443-9.
  http://www.ncbi.nlm.nih.gov:80/entrez/query.fcgi?cmd=Retrieve&db=
  PubMed&list_uids=2432797&dopt=Abstract

- **Neurophysiological and neuroradiological features preceding infantile spasms.**
  Author(s): Watanabe K, Takeuchi T, Hakamada S, Hayakawa F.
  Source: Brain & Development. 1987; 9(4): 391-8.
  http://www.ncbi.nlm.nih.gov:80/entrez/query.fcgi?cmd=Retrieve&db=
  PubMed&list_uids=3434714&dopt=Abstract

- **Neuroradiological aspects of infantile spasms.**
  Author(s): Ludwig B.
  Source: Brain & Development. 1987; 9(4): 358-60. Review.
  http://www.ncbi.nlm.nih.gov:80/entrez/query.fcgi?cmd=Retrieve&db=
  PubMed&list_uids=3324793&dopt=Abstract

- **Neurosteroids and infantile spasms: the deoxycorticosterone hypothesis.**
  Author(s): Rogawski MA, Reddy DS.
  Source: Int Rev Neurobiol. 2002; 49: 199-219. Review.
  http://www.ncbi.nlm.nih.gov:80/entrez/query.fcgi?cmd=Retrieve&db=
  PubMed&list_uids=12040893&dopt=Abstract

- **Newer GABAergic agents for pharmacotherapy of infantile spasms.**
  Author(s): Reddy DS.
  Source: Drugs Today (Barc). 2002 October; 38(10): 657-75. Review.
  http://www.ncbi.nlm.nih.gov:80/entrez/query.fcgi?cmd=Retrieve&db=
  PubMed&list_uids=12582452&dopt=Abstract

- **Nitrazepam for refractory infantile spasms and the Lennox-Gastaut syndrome.**
  Author(s): Chamberlain MC.
  Source: Journal of Child Neurology. 1996 January; 11(1): 31-4.
  http://www.ncbi.nlm.nih.gov:80/entrez/query.fcgi?cmd=Retrieve&db=
  PubMed&list_uids=8745382&dopt=Abstract

- **Nodding attacks (infantile spasms) associated with temporal lobe astrocytoma--case report.**
  Author(s): Morimoto K, Abekura M, Nii Y, Nakatani S, Hayakawa T, Mogami H.
  Source: Neurol Med Chir (Tokyo). 1989 July; 29(7): 610-3.
  http://www.ncbi.nlm.nih.gov:80/entrez/query.fcgi?cmd=Retrieve&db=
  PubMed&list_uids=2477762&dopt=Abstract

- **Non-verbal communication skills of surgically treated children with infantile spasms.**
  Author(s): Caplan R, Guthrie D, Mundy P, Sigman M, Shields D, Sherman T, Peacock WJ.
  Source: Developmental Medicine and Child Neurology. 1992 June; 34(6): 499-506.
  http://www.ncbi.nlm.nih.gov:80/entrez/query.fcgi?cmd=Retrieve&db=
  PubMed&list_uids=1377138&dopt=Abstract

- **Occurrence, outcome, and prognostic factors of infantile spasms and Lennox-Gastaut syndrome.**
  Author(s): Rantala H, Putkonen T.
  Source: Epilepsia. 1999 March; 40(3): 286-9.
  http://www.ncbi.nlm.nih.gov:80/entrez/query.fcgi?cmd=Retrieve&db=PubMed&list_uids=10080506&dopt=Abstract

- **Oral high-dose phenobarbital therapy for early infantile epileptic encephalopathy.**
  Author(s): Ozawa H, Kawada Y, Noma S, Sugai K.
  Source: Pediatric Neurology. 2002 March; 26(3): 222-4.
  http://www.ncbi.nlm.nih.gov:80/entrez/query.fcgi?cmd=Retrieve&db=PubMed&list_uids=11955931&dopt=Abstract

- **Overnight polygraphic studies of infantile spasms--influence of hormone therapy on sleep states, pulse, respiration and seizure activities.**
  Author(s): Horita H, Hoashi E, Okuyama Y, Kumagai K, Endo S.
  Source: Folia Psychiatr Neurol Jpn. 1979; 33(3): 268-77.
  http://www.ncbi.nlm.nih.gov:80/entrez/query.fcgi?cmd=Retrieve&db=PubMed&list_uids=230134&dopt=Abstract

- **Overnight polygraphic study of agenesis of the corpus callosum with seizures resembling infantile spasms.**
  Author(s): Horita H, Kumagai K, Maekawa K, Endo S.
  Source: Brain & Development. 1980; 2(4): 379-86.
  http://www.ncbi.nlm.nih.gov:80/entrez/query.fcgi?cmd=Retrieve&db=PubMed&list_uids=6261603&dopt=Abstract

- **Partial seizures evolving to infantile spasms.**
  Author(s): Yamamoto N, Watanabe K, Negoro T, Furune S, Takahashi I, Nomura K, Matsumoto A.
  Source: Epilepsia. 1988 January-February; 29(1): 34-40.
  http://www.ncbi.nlm.nih.gov:80/entrez/query.fcgi?cmd=Retrieve&db=PubMed&list_uids=3123212&dopt=Abstract

- **Pathophysiology of infantile spasms.**
  Author(s): Chugani HT.
  Source: Advances in Experimental Medicine and Biology. 2002; 497: 111-21. Review.
  http://www.ncbi.nlm.nih.gov:80/entrez/query.fcgi?cmd=Retrieve&db=PubMed&list_uids=11993727&dopt=Abstract

- **Pathophysiology of massive infantile spasms: perspective on the putative role of the brain adrenal axis.**
  Author(s): Baram TZ.
  Source: Annals of Neurology. 1993 March; 33(3): 231-6. Review.
  http://www.ncbi.nlm.nih.gov:80/entrez/query.fcgi?cmd=Retrieve&db=PubMed&list_uids=8388675&dopt=Abstract

- **Pattern reversal evoked potentials in infantile spasms.**
  Author(s): Taddeucci G, Fiorentini A, Pirchio M, Spinelli D.
  Source: Hum Neurobiol. 1984; 3(3): 153-5.
  http://www.ncbi.nlm.nih.gov:80/entrez/query.fcgi?cmd=Retrieve&db=PubMed&list_uids=6480435&dopt=Abstract

- **Phasic motor activity reduction occurring with horizontal rapid eye movements during REM sleep is disturbed in infantile spasms.**
  Author(s): Kohyama J, Ohsawa Y, Shimohira M, Iwakawa Y.
  Source: Journal of the Neurological Sciences. 1996 June; 138(1-2): 82-7.
  http://www.ncbi.nlm.nih.gov:80/entrez/query.fcgi?cmd=Retrieve&db=PubMed&list_uids=8791243&dopt=Abstract

- **Pneumocystis carinii pneumonia associated with adrenocorticotropic hormone treatment for infantile spasms.**
  Author(s): Shamir R, Garty BZ.
  Source: European Journal of Pediatrics. 1992 November; 151(11): 867.
  http://www.ncbi.nlm.nih.gov:80/entrez/query.fcgi?cmd=Retrieve&db=PubMed&list_uids=1468469&dopt=Abstract

- **Pneumocystis carinii pneumonia in a child receiving ACTH for infantile spasms.**
  Author(s): Dunagan DP, Rubin BK, Fasano MB.
  Source: Pediatric Pulmonology. 1999 April; 27(4): 286-9. Review.
  http://www.ncbi.nlm.nih.gov:80/entrez/query.fcgi?cmd=Retrieve&db=PubMed&list_uids=10230930&dopt=Abstract

- **Pneumocystis carinii pneumonia in infants given adrenocorticotropic hormone for infantile spasms.**
  Author(s): Quittell LM, Fisher M, Foley CM.
  Source: The Journal of Pediatrics. 1987 June; 110(6): 901-3.
  http://www.ncbi.nlm.nih.gov:80/entrez/query.fcgi?cmd=Retrieve&db=PubMed&list_uids=3035157&dopt=Abstract

- **Pneumoencephalographic and EEG observations in 106 children with infantile spasms.**
  Author(s): Harris R, Hoare RD, Crichton JU, Pampiglione G.
  Source: Electroencephalography and Clinical Neurophysiology. 1967 April; 22(4): 394.
  http://www.ncbi.nlm.nih.gov:80/entrez/query.fcgi?cmd=Retrieve&db=PubMed&list_uids=4164762&dopt=Abstract

- **Pneumonia in infants given adrenocorticotropic hormone for infantile spasms.**
  Author(s): Lopez Aguado J, Greaves T, Hutchison HT, McCarty JM.
  Source: The Journal of Pediatrics. 1988 March; 112(3): 508.
  http://www.ncbi.nlm.nih.gov:80/entrez/query.fcgi?cmd=Retrieve&db=PubMed&list_uids=2831332&dopt=Abstract

- **Polygraphic study during whole night sleep in infantile spasms.**
  Author(s): Fukuyama Y, Shionaga A, Iida Y.
  Source: European Neurology. 1979; 18(5): 302-11.
  http://www.ncbi.nlm.nih.gov:80/entrez/query.fcgi?cmd=Retrieve&db=PubMed&list_uids=230967&dopt=Abstract

- **Posterior fossa abnormalities in children with infantile spasms.**
  Author(s): Schiffmann R, Mannheim GB, Stafstrom CE, Hamburger SD, Holmes GL.
  Source: Journal of Child Neurology. 1993 October; 8(4): 360-5.
  http://www.ncbi.nlm.nih.gov:80/entrez/query.fcgi?cmd=Retrieve&db=PubMed&list_uids=7693798&dopt=Abstract

- **Precise characterization and quantification of infantile spasms.**
  Author(s): Kellaway P, Hrachovy RA, Frost JD Jr, Zion T.
  Source: Annals of Neurology. 1979 September; 6(3): 214-8.
  http://www.ncbi.nlm.nih.gov:80/entrez/query.fcgi?cmd=Retrieve&db=PubMed&list_uids=534418&dopt=Abstract

- **Prognosis for seizure control in infantile spasms preceded by other seizures.**
  Author(s): Velez A, Dulac O, Plouin P.
  Source: Brain & Development. 1990; 12(3): 306-9.
  http://www.ncbi.nlm.nih.gov:80/entrez/query.fcgi?cmd=Retrieve&db=PubMed&list_uids=2403200&dopt=Abstract

- **Prognosis of infantile spasms.**
  Author(s): Chevrie JJ.
  Source: The Journal of Pediatrics. 1982 October; 101(4): 650-1.
  http://www.ncbi.nlm.nih.gov:80/entrez/query.fcgi?cmd=Retrieve&db=PubMed&list_uids=7119978&dopt=Abstract

- **Prognostic factors of infantile spasms from the etiological viewpoint.**
  Author(s): Matsumoto A, Watanabe K, Negoro T, Sugiura M, Iwase K, Hara K, Miyazaki S.
  Source: Brain & Development. 1981; 3(4): 361-4.
  http://www.ncbi.nlm.nih.gov:80/entrez/query.fcgi?cmd=Retrieve&db=PubMed&list_uids=6274214&dopt=Abstract

- **Progressive generalized brain atrophy and infantile spasms associated with cytochrome c oxidase deficiency.**
  Author(s): Bakker HD, Van den Bogert C, Drewes JG, Barth PG, Scholte HR, Wanders RJ, Ruitenbeek W.
  Source: Journal of Inherited Metabolic Disease. 1996; 19(2): 153-6.
  http://www.ncbi.nlm.nih.gov:80/entrez/query.fcgi?cmd=Retrieve&db=PubMed&list_uids=8739953&dopt=Abstract

- **Prolactin levels in cerebrospinal fluid of patients with infantile spasms.**
  Author(s): Aydln GB, Kose G, Degerliyurt A, Din N, Camurdanoglu D, Cakmak F.
  Source: Pediatric Neurology. 2002 October; 27(4): 267-70.
  http://www.ncbi.nlm.nih.gov:80/entrez/query.fcgi?cmd=Retrieve&db=PubMed&list_uids=12435564&dopt=Abstract

- **Prospective preliminary analysis of the development of autism and epilepsy in children with infantile spasms.**
  Author(s): Askalan R, Mackay M, Brian J, Otsubo H, McDermott C, Bryson S, Boyd J, Snead C 3rd, Roberts W, Weiss S.
  Source: Journal of Child Neurology. 2003 March; 18(3): 165-70.
  http://www.ncbi.nlm.nih.gov:80/entrez/query.fcgi?cmd=Retrieve&db=PubMed&list_uids=12731640&dopt=Abstract

- **Prospective study of outcome of infants with infantile spasms treated during controlled studies of ACTH and prednisone.**
  Author(s): Glaze DG, Hrachovy RA, Frost JD Jr, Kellaway P, Zion TE.
  Source: The Journal of Pediatrics. 1988 March; 112(3): 389-96.
  http://www.ncbi.nlm.nih.gov:80/entrez/query.fcgi?cmd=Retrieve&db=PubMed&list_uids=2450190&dopt=Abstract

- **Psychiatric disorders following infantile spasms.**
  Author(s): Thornton EM, Pampiglione G.
  Source: Lancet. 1979 June 16; 1(8129): 1297.
  http://www.ncbi.nlm.nih.gov:80/entrez/query.fcgi?cmd=Retrieve&db=PubMed&list_uids=87760&dopt=Abstract

- **Psychiatric disorders in children with earlier infantile spasms.**
  Author(s): Riikonen R, Amnell G.
  Source: Developmental Medicine and Child Neurology. 1981 December; 23(6): 747-60.
  http://www.ncbi.nlm.nih.gov:80/entrez/query.fcgi?cmd=Retrieve&db=PubMed&list_uids=7319142&dopt=Abstract

- **Putative neurotransmitter abnormalities in infantile spasms: cerebrospinal fluid neurochemistry and drug effects.**
  Author(s): Pranzatelli MR.
  Source: Journal of Child Neurology. 1994 April; 9(2): 119-29. Review.
  http://www.ncbi.nlm.nih.gov:80/entrez/query.fcgi?cmd=Retrieve&db=PubMed&list_uids=7911815&dopt=Abstract

- **Pyridoxine therapy on Nigerian children with infantile spasms.**
  Author(s): Izuora GI, Iloeje SO.
  Source: East Afr Med J. 1989 August; 66(8): 525-30.
  http://www.ncbi.nlm.nih.gov:80/entrez/query.fcgi?cmd=Retrieve&db=PubMed&list_uids=2606037&dopt=Abstract

- **Pyruvate carboxylase deficiency: acute exacerbation after ACTH treatment of infantile spasms.**
  Author(s): Rutledge SL, Snead OC 3rd, Kelly DR, Kerr DS, Swann JW, Spink DL, Martin DL.
  Source: Pediatric Neurology. 1989 July-August; 5(4): 249-52.
  http://www.ncbi.nlm.nih.gov:80/entrez/query.fcgi?cmd=Retrieve&db=PubMed&list_uids=2553027&dopt=Abstract

- **Quantitative analysis and characterization of infantile spasms.**
  Author(s): Frost JD Jr, Hrachovy RA, Kellaway P, Zion T.
  Source: Epilepsia. 1978 June; 19(3): 273-82.
  http://www.ncbi.nlm.nih.gov:80/entrez/query.fcgi?cmd=Retrieve&db=PubMed&list_uids=679895&dopt=Abstract

- **Randomised, placebo-controlled study of vigabatrin as first-line treatment of infantile spasms.**
  Author(s): Appleton RE, Peters AC, Mumford JP, Shaw DE.
  Source: Epilepsia. 1999 November; 40(11): 1627-33.
  http://www.ncbi.nlm.nih.gov:80/entrez/query.fcgi?cmd=Retrieve&db=PubMed&list_uids=10565592&dopt=Abstract

- **Randomized trial comparing vigabatrin and hydrocortisone in infantile spasms due to tuberous sclerosis.**
  Author(s): Chiron C, Dumas C, Jambaque I, Mumford J, Dulac O.
  Source: Epilepsy Research. 1997 January; 26(2): 389-95.
  http://www.ncbi.nlm.nih.gov:80/entrez/query.fcgi?cmd=Retrieve&db=PubMed&list_uids=9095401&dopt=Abstract

- **Randomized trial of vigabatrin in patients with infantile spasms.**
  Author(s): Lux AL, Edwards SW, Osborne JP, Hancock E, Johnson AL, Verity CM, Kennedy CR, O'Callaghan FJ, Newton RW.
  Source: Neurology. 2002 August 27; 59(4): 648.
  http://www.ncbi.nlm.nih.gov:80/entrez/query.fcgi?cmd=Retrieve&db=PubMed&list_uids=12196676&dopt=Abstract

- **Randomized trial of vigabatrin in patients with infantile spasms.**
  Author(s): Elterman RD, Shields WD, Mansfield KA, Nakagawa J; US Infantile Spasms Vigabatrin Study Group.
  Source: Neurology. 2001 October 23; 57(8): 1416-21.
  http://www.ncbi.nlm.nih.gov:80/entrez/query.fcgi?cmd=Retrieve&db=PubMed&list_uids=11673582&dopt=Abstract

- **Rapid enlargement of cardiac rhabdomyoma during corticotropin therapy for infantile spasms.**
  Author(s): Hishitani T, Hoshino K, Ogawa K, Uehara R, Kitazawa R, Hamano S, Nara T, Ogawa Y.
  Source: The Canadian Journal of Cardiology. 1997 January; 13(1): 72-4.
  http://www.ncbi.nlm.nih.gov:80/entrez/query.fcgi?cmd=Retrieve&db=PubMed&list_uids=9039068&dopt=Abstract

- **Reappraisal of interictal electroencephalograms in infantile spasms.**
  Author(s): Watanabe K, Negoro T, Aso K, Matsumoto A.
  Source: Epilepsia. 1993 July-August; 34(4): 679-85.
  http://www.ncbi.nlm.nih.gov:80/entrez/query.fcgi?cmd=Retrieve&db=PubMed&list_uids=8330578&dopt=Abstract

- **Recent advances in infantile spasms research in Finland.**
  Author(s): Riikonen R.
  Source: Acta Paediatr Jpn. 1987 February; 29(1): 70-6. Review. No Abstract Available.
  http://www.ncbi.nlm.nih.gov:80/entrez/query.fcgi?cmd=Retrieve&db=PubMed&list_uids=2849853&dopt=Abstract

- **Reduced ACTH content in cerebrospinal fluid of children affected by cryptogenic infantile spasms with hypsarrhythmia.**
  Author(s): Nalin A, Facchinetti F, Galli V, Petraglia F, Storchi R, Genazzani AR.
  Source: Epilepsia. 1985 September-October; 26(5): 446-9.
  http://www.ncbi.nlm.nih.gov:80/entrez/query.fcgi?cmd=Retrieve&db=PubMed&list_uids=2995025&dopt=Abstract

- **REM sleep components predict the response to initial treatment of infantile spasms.**
  Author(s): Kohyama J, Sugimoto J, Itoh M, Sakuma H, Shimohira M, Hasegawa T, Iwakawa Y.
  Source: Epilepsia. 1999 July; 40(7): 992-6.
  http://www.ncbi.nlm.nih.gov:80/entrez/query.fcgi?cmd=Retrieve&db=PubMed&list_uids=10403225&dopt=Abstract

- **Renal and pancreatic calcification during treatment of infantile spasms with ACTH.**
  Author(s): Hanefeld F, Sperner J, Rating D, Rausch H, Kaufmann HJ.
  Source: Lancet. 1984 April 21; 1(8382): 901.
  http://www.ncbi.nlm.nih.gov:80/entrez/query.fcgi?cmd=Retrieve&db=PubMed&list_uids=6143199&dopt=Abstract

- **Respiratory chain complex I deficiency in an infant with infantile spasms.**
  Author(s): Verdu A, Alonso LA, Arenas J.
  Source: Journal of Neurology, Neurosurgery, and Psychiatry. 1996 March; 60(3): 349.
  http://www.ncbi.nlm.nih.gov:80/entrez/query.fcgi?cmd=Retrieve&db=PubMed&list_uids=8609522&dopt=Abstract

- **Results of treatment and clinico-electroencephalographic evolution of infantile spasms.**
  Author(s): Wiszczor-Adamczyk B, Koslacz-Folga A.
  Source: Pol Med J. 1969; 8(1): 193-9. No Abstract Available.
  http://www.ncbi.nlm.nih.gov:80/entrez/query.fcgi?cmd=Retrieve&db=PubMed&list_uids=4305685&dopt=Abstract

- **Reversible cerebral atrophy in infantile spasms caused by corticotrophin.**
  Author(s): Lyen KR, Holland IM, Lyen YC.
  Source: Lancet. 1979 July 7; 2(8132): 37-8.
  http://www.ncbi.nlm.nih.gov:80/entrez/query.fcgi?cmd=Retrieve&db=PubMed&list_uids=87909&dopt=Abstract

- **Revised guideline for prescribing vigabatrin in children. Guideline's claim about infantile spasms is not based on appropriate evidence.**
  Author(s): Lux AL, Edwards SW, Osborne JP, Hancock E, Johnson AL, Kennedy CR, O'Callaghan FJ, Newton RW, Verity CM.
  Source: Bmj (Clinical Research Ed.). 2001 January 27; 322(7280): 236-7.
  http://www.ncbi.nlm.nih.gov:80/entrez/query.fcgi?cmd=Retrieve&db=PubMed&list_uids=11159628&dopt=Abstract

- **Risk factors associated with infantile spasms: a hospital-based case-control study in Taiwan.**
  Author(s): Liou HH, Oon PC, Lin HC, Wang PJ, Chen TH.
  Source: Epilepsy Research. 2001 November; 47(1-2): 91-8.
  http://www.ncbi.nlm.nih.gov:80/entrez/query.fcgi?cmd=Retrieve&db=PubMed&list_uids=11673024&dopt=Abstract

- **Risk factors of infantile spasms compared with other seizures in children under 2 years of age.**
  Author(s): Rantala H, Shields WD, Christenson PD, Nielsen C, Buch D, Jacobsen V, Zachau-Christiansen B, Uhari M, Cherry JD.
  Source: Epilepsia. 1996 April; 37(4): 362-6.
  http://www.ncbi.nlm.nih.gov:80/entrez/query.fcgi?cmd=Retrieve&db=PubMed&list_uids=8603641&dopt=Abstract

- **Risk of infection during adrenocorticotropic hormone treatment in infants with infantile spasms.**
  Author(s): Shamir R, Garty BZ, Rachmel A, Kivity S, Alpert G.
  Source: The Pediatric Infectious Disease Journal. 1993 November; 12(11): 913-6.
  http://www.ncbi.nlm.nih.gov:80/entrez/query.fcgi?cmd=Retrieve&db=PubMed&list_uids=8265280&dopt=Abstract

- **Role of subcortical structures in the pathogenesis of infantile spasms: what are possible subcortical mediators?**
  Author(s): Lado FA, Moshe SL.
  Source: Int Rev Neurobiol. 2002; 49: 115-40. Review.
  http://www.ncbi.nlm.nih.gov:80/entrez/query.fcgi?cmd=Retrieve&db=PubMed&list_uids=12040889&dopt=Abstract

- **Septo-optic dysplasia with infantile spasms.**
  Author(s): Kuriyama M, Shigematsu Y, Konishi K, Konishi Y, Sudo M, Haruki S, Ito H.
  Source: Pediatric Neurology. 1988 January-February; 4(1): 62-5.
  http://www.ncbi.nlm.nih.gov:80/entrez/query.fcgi?cmd=Retrieve&db=PubMed&list_uids=3233109&dopt=Abstract

- **Sequential CT studies of 24 children with infantile spasms on ACTH therapy.**
  Author(s): Ito M, Takao T, Okuno T, Mikawa H.
  Source: Developmental Medicine and Child Neurology. 1983 August; 25(4): 475-80.
  http://www.ncbi.nlm.nih.gov:80/entrez/query.fcgi?cmd=Retrieve&db=PubMed&list_uids=6311654&dopt=Abstract

- **Serologic HLA typing in infantile spasms.**
  Author(s): Hrachovy RA, Frost JD Jr, Pollack MS, Glaze DG.
  Source: Epilepsia. 1988 November-December; 29(6): 817-9.
  http://www.ncbi.nlm.nih.gov:80/entrez/query.fcgi?cmd=Retrieve&db=PubMed&list_uids=3191897&dopt=Abstract

- **Serum steroids and success of corticotropin therapy in infantile spasms.**
  Author(s): Riikonen R, Perheentupa J.
  Source: Acta Paediatr Scand. 1986 July; 75(4): 598-600.
  http://www.ncbi.nlm.nih.gov:80/entrez/query.fcgi?cmd=Retrieve&db=PubMed&list_uids=3019075&dopt=Abstract

- **Short term effects of valproate on infantile spasms.**
  Author(s): Dyken PR, DuRant RH, Minden DB, King DW.
  Source: Pediatric Neurology. 1985 January-February; 1(1): 34-7.
  http://www.ncbi.nlm.nih.gov:80/entrez/query.fcgi?cmd=Retrieve&db=PubMed&list_uids=3939740&dopt=Abstract

- **Simultaneous infantile spasms and partial seizures.**
  Author(s): Donat JF, Wright FS.
  Source: Journal of Child Neurology. 1991 July; 6(3): 246-50.
  http://www.ncbi.nlm.nih.gov:80/entrez/query.fcgi?cmd=Retrieve&db=PubMed&list_uids=1875027&dopt=Abstract

- **Sleep characteristics in infantile spasms.**
  Author(s): Hrachovy RA, Frost JD Jr, Kellaway P.
  Source: Neurology. 1981 June; 31(6): 688-93.
  http://www.ncbi.nlm.nih.gov:80/entrez/query.fcgi?cmd=Retrieve&db=PubMed&list_uids=6264348&dopt=Abstract

- **Some aspects of infantile spasms.**
  Author(s): Soetomenggolo TS, Purboyo RH, Hendarto SK, Ismael S.
  Source: Paediatr Indones. 1986 September-October; 26(9-10): 165-76. No Abstract Available.
  http://www.ncbi.nlm.nih.gov:80/entrez/query.fcgi?cmd=Retrieve&db=PubMed&list_uids=3808734&dopt=Abstract

- **Spectral properties of EEG fast activity ictal discharges associated with infantile spasms.**
  Author(s): Panzica F, Franceschetti S, Binelli S, Canafoglia L, Granata T, Avanzini G.
  Source: Clinical Neurophysiology : Official Journal of the International Federation of Clinical Neurophysiology. 1999 April; 110(4): 593-603.
  http://www.ncbi.nlm.nih.gov:80/entrez/query.fcgi?cmd=Retrieve&db=PubMed&list_uids=10378727&dopt=Abstract

- **Spontaneous remission of infantile spasms with hypsarhythmia.**
  Author(s): Bachman DS.
  Source: Archives of Neurology. 1981 December; 38(12): 785.
  http://www.ncbi.nlm.nih.gov:80/entrez/query.fcgi?cmd=Retrieve&db=PubMed&list_uids=7316851&dopt=Abstract

- **Steroid treatment of infantile spasms with hypsarrhythmia.**
  Author(s): Oftedal SI.
  Source: Electroencephalography and Clinical Neurophysiology. 1967 October; 23(4): 390-1.
  http://www.ncbi.nlm.nih.gov:80/entrez/query.fcgi?cmd=Retrieve&db=PubMed&list_uids=4167812&dopt=Abstract

- **Steroids or vigabatrin in the treatment of infantile spasms?**
  Author(s): Riikonen RS.
  Source: Pediatric Neurology. 2000 November; 23(5): 403-8. Review.
  http://www.ncbi.nlm.nih.gov:80/entrez/query.fcgi?cmd=Retrieve&db=PubMed&list_uids=11118795&dopt=Abstract

- **Studies on CSF tryptophan metabolism in infantile spasms.**
  Author(s): Yamamoto H.
  Source: Pediatric Neurology. 1991 November-December; 7(6): 411-4.
  http://www.ncbi.nlm.nih.gov:80/entrez/query.fcgi?cmd=Retrieve&db=PubMed&list_uids=1724601&dopt=Abstract

- **Suppressed pituitary ACTH response after ACTH treatment of infantile spasms.**
  Author(s): Ross DL.
  Source: Journal of Child Neurology. 1986 January; 1(1): 34-7.
  http://www.ncbi.nlm.nih.gov:80/entrez/query.fcgi?cmd=Retrieve&db=
  PubMed&list_uids=3036933&dopt=Abstract

- **Suppressive action of ACTH on growth hormone secretion in patients with infantile spasms.**
  Author(s): Izumi T, Imaizumi C, Ashida E, Ochiai T, Wang PJ, Fukuyama Y.
  Source: Brain & Development. 1985; 7(6): 636-9.
  http://www.ncbi.nlm.nih.gov:80/entrez/query.fcgi?cmd=Retrieve&db=
  PubMed&list_uids=3008584&dopt=Abstract

- **Surgery for intractable infantile spasms: neuroimaging perspectives.**
  Author(s): Chugani HT, Shewmon DA, Shields WD, Sankar R, Comair Y, Vinters HV, Peacock WJ.
  Source: Epilepsia. 1993 July-August; 34(4): 764-71.
  http://www.ncbi.nlm.nih.gov:80/entrez/query.fcgi?cmd=Retrieve&db=
  PubMed&list_uids=8330590&dopt=Abstract

- **Surgery for the treatment of medically intractable infantile spasms: a cautionary case.**
  Author(s): Shields WD, Shewmon DA, Peacock WJ, LoPresti CM, Nakagawa JA, Yudovin S.
  Source: Epilepsia. 1999 September; 40(9): 1305-8.
  http://www.ncbi.nlm.nih.gov:80/entrez/query.fcgi?cmd=Retrieve&db=
  PubMed&list_uids=10487196&dopt=Abstract

- **Surgical treatment for infantile spasms?**
  Author(s): Hrachovy RA, Frost JD Jr, Glaze DG, Kellaway P.
  Source: Annals of Neurology. 1991 January; 29(1): 110-2.
  http://www.ncbi.nlm.nih.gov:80/entrez/query.fcgi?cmd=Retrieve&db=
  PubMed&list_uids=1996874&dopt=Abstract

- **Symptomatology of infantile spasms.**
  Author(s): Watanabe K, Negoro T, Okumura A.
  Source: Brain & Development. 2001 November; 23(7): 453-66. Review.
  http://www.ncbi.nlm.nih.gov:80/entrez/query.fcgi?cmd=Retrieve&db=
  PubMed&list_uids=11701239&dopt=Abstract

- **Temporal relationship modeling: DTP or DT immunizations and infantile spasms.**
  Author(s): Goodman M, Lamm SH, Bellman MH.
  Source: Vaccine. 1998 January-February; 16(2-3): 225-31.
  http://www.ncbi.nlm.nih.gov:80/entrez/query.fcgi?cmd=Retrieve&db=PubMed&list_uids=9607034&dopt=Abstract

- **The descriptive epidemiology of infantile spasms among Atlanta children.**
  Author(s): Trevathan E, Murphy CC, Yeargin-Allsopp M.
  Source: Epilepsia. 1999 June; 40(6): 748-51.
  http://www.ncbi.nlm.nih.gov:80/entrez/query.fcgi?cmd=Retrieve&db=PubMed&list_uids=10368073&dopt=Abstract

- **The effect of non-depot ACTH(1-24) on infantile spasms.**
  Author(s): Kusse MC, van Nieuwenhuizen O, van Huffelen AC, van der Mey W, Thijssen JH, van Ree JM.
  Source: Developmental Medicine and Child Neurology. 1993 December; 35(12): 1067-73.
  http://www.ncbi.nlm.nih.gov:80/entrez/query.fcgi?cmd=Retrieve&db=PubMed&list_uids=8253287&dopt=Abstract

- **The epidemiology of infantile spasms.**
  Author(s): Brna PM, Gordon KE, Dooley JM, Wood EP.
  Source: The Canadian Journal of Neurological Sciences. Le Journal Canadien Des Sciences Neurologiques. 2001 November; 28(4): 309-12.
  http://www.ncbi.nlm.nih.gov:80/entrez/query.fcgi?cmd=Retrieve&db=PubMed&list_uids=11766774&dopt=Abstract

- **The treatment of infantile spasms by child neurologists.**
  Author(s): Bobele GB, Bodensteiner JB.
  Source: Journal of Child Neurology. 1994 October; 9(4): 432-5.
  http://www.ncbi.nlm.nih.gov:80/entrez/query.fcgi?cmd=Retrieve&db=PubMed&list_uids=7822738&dopt=Abstract

- **The treatment of infantile spasms by paediatric neurologists in the UK and Ireland.**
  Author(s): Appleton RE.
  Source: Developmental Medicine and Child Neurology. 1996 March; 38(3): 278-9.
  http://www.ncbi.nlm.nih.gov:80/entrez/query.fcgi?cmd=Retrieve&db=PubMed&list_uids=8631525&dopt=Abstract

- **The use of felbamate to treat infantile spasms.**
  Author(s): Stafstrom CE.
  Source: Journal of Child Neurology. 1996 March; 11(2): 170-1.
  http://www.ncbi.nlm.nih.gov:80/entrez/query.fcgi?cmd=Retrieve&db=
  PubMed&list_uids=8881998&dopt=Abstract

- **The use of felbamate to treat infantile spasms.**
  Author(s): Hurst DL, Rolan TD.
  Source: Journal of Child Neurology. 1995 March; 10(2): 134-6.
  http://www.ncbi.nlm.nih.gov:80/entrez/query.fcgi?cmd=Retrieve&db=
  PubMed&list_uids=7782604&dopt=Abstract

- **The use of vigabatrin in infantile spasms in Asian children.**
  Author(s): Tay SK, Ong HT, Low PS.
  Source: Ann Acad Med Singapore. 2001 January; 30(1): 26-31.
  http://www.ncbi.nlm.nih.gov:80/entrez/query.fcgi?cmd=Retrieve&db=
  PubMed&list_uids=11242620&dopt=Abstract

- **The X-linked infantile spasms syndrome (MIM 308350) maps to Xp11.4-Xpter in two pedigrees.**
  Author(s): Claes S, Devriendt K, Lagae L, Ceulemans B, Dom L, Casaer P, Raeymaekers P, Cassiman JJ, Fryns JP.
  Source: Annals of Neurology. 1997 September; 42(3): 360-4.
  http://www.ncbi.nlm.nih.gov:80/entrez/query.fcgi?cmd=Retrieve&db=
  PubMed&list_uids=9307258&dopt=Abstract

- **Therapeutic efficacy of ACTH in symptomatic infantile spasms with hypsarrhythmia.**
  Author(s): Sher PK, Sheikh MR.
  Source: Pediatric Neurology. 1993 November-December; 9(6): 451-6.
  http://www.ncbi.nlm.nih.gov:80/entrez/query.fcgi?cmd=Retrieve&db=
  PubMed&list_uids=7605553&dopt=Abstract

- **Treatment of infantile spasms with high-dosage vitamin B6.**
  Author(s): Pietz J, Benninger C, Schafer H, Sontheimer D, Mittermaier G, Rating D.
  Source: Epilepsia. 1993 July-August; 34(4): 757-63.
  http://www.ncbi.nlm.nih.gov:80/entrez/query.fcgi?cmd=Retrieve&db=
  PubMed&list_uids=8330589&dopt=Abstract

- **Treatment of infantile spasms with high-dose oral prednisolone.**
  Author(s): Hancock E, Osborne J.
  Source: Developmental Medicine and Child Neurology. 1998 July; 40(7): 500.
  http://www.ncbi.nlm.nih.gov:80/entrez/query.fcgi?cmd=Retrieve&db=PubMed&list_uids=9698065&dopt=Abstract

- **Treatment of infantile spasms with zonisamide.**
  Author(s): Yanai S, Hanai T, Narazaki O.
  Source: Brain & Development. 1999 April; 21(3): 157-61.
  http://www.ncbi.nlm.nih.gov:80/entrez/query.fcgi?cmd=Retrieve&db=PubMed&list_uids=10372900&dopt=Abstract

- **Treatment of infantile spasms.**
  Author(s): Hancock E, Osborne J, Milner P.
  Source: Cochrane Database Syst Rev. 2003; (3): Cd001770. Review.
  http://www.ncbi.nlm.nih.gov:80/entrez/query.fcgi?cmd=Retrieve&db=PubMed&list_uids=12917912&dopt=Abstract

- **Treatment of infantile spasms.**
  Author(s): Hancock E, Osborne JP, Milner P.
  Source: Cochrane Database Syst Rev. 2002; (2): Cd001770. Review. Update In:
  http://www.ncbi.nlm.nih.gov:80/entrez/query.fcgi?cmd=Retrieve&db=PubMed&list_uids=12076419&dopt=Abstract

- **Treatment of infantile spasms.**
  Author(s): Haines ST, Casto DT.
  Source: The Annals of Pharmacotherapy. 1994 June; 28(6): 779-91. Review.
  http://www.ncbi.nlm.nih.gov:80/entrez/query.fcgi?cmd=Retrieve&db=PubMed&list_uids=7919570&dopt=Abstract

- **Treatment of infantile spasms: an evidence-based approach.**
  Author(s): Mackay M, Weiss S, Snead OC 3rd.
  Source: Int Rev Neurobiol. 2002; 49: 157-84. Review.
  http://www.ncbi.nlm.nih.gov:80/entrez/query.fcgi?cmd=Retrieve&db=PubMed&list_uids=12040891&dopt=Abstract

- **Treatment of infantile spasms: results of a population-based study with vigabatrin as the first drug for spasms.**
  Author(s): Granstrom ML, Gaily E, Liukkonen E.
  Source: Epilepsia. 1999 July; 40(7): 950-7.
  http://www.ncbi.nlm.nih.gov:80/entrez/query.fcgi?cmd=Retrieve&db=PubMed&list_uids=10403219&dopt=Abstract

- **Treatment of infantile spasms: the ideal and the mundane.**
  Author(s): Baram TZ.
  Source: Epilepsia. 2003 August; 44(8): 993-4.
  http://www.ncbi.nlm.nih.gov:80/entrez/query.fcgi?cmd=Retrieve&db=PubMed&list_uids=12887429&dopt=Abstract

- **Unilateral hemispheric ganglioglioma with infantile spasms.**
  Author(s): Gabriel YH.
  Source: Annals of Neurology. 1980 March; 7(3): 287-8.
  http://www.ncbi.nlm.nih.gov:80/entrez/query.fcgi?cmd=Retrieve&db=PubMed&list_uids=7425564&dopt=Abstract

- **Unilateral porencephalic cyst presenting as infantile spasms: a case report.**
  Author(s): Ou SF, Chi CS, Shian WJ, Mak SC, Wong TT.
  Source: Zhonghua Yi Xue Za Zhi (Taipei). 1995 February; 55(2): 203-8.
  http://www.ncbi.nlm.nih.gov:80/entrez/query.fcgi?cmd=Retrieve&db=PubMed&list_uids=7750065&dopt=Abstract

- **Unusual variants of infantile spasms.**
  Author(s): Donat JF, Wright FS.
  Source: Journal of Child Neurology. 1991 October; 6(4): 313-8.
  http://www.ncbi.nlm.nih.gov:80/entrez/query.fcgi?cmd=Retrieve&db=PubMed&list_uids=1940132&dopt=Abstract

- **Use of ACTH fragments of children with infantile spasms.**
  Author(s): Willig RP, Lagenstein I.
  Source: Neuropediatrics. 1982 May; 13(2): 55-8.
  http://www.ncbi.nlm.nih.gov:80/entrez/query.fcgi?cmd=Retrieve&db=PubMed&list_uids=6290926&dopt=Abstract

- **Use of valproic acid in treatment of infantile spasms.**
  Author(s): Bachman DS.
  Source: Archives of Neurology. 1982 January; 39(1): 49-52.
  http://www.ncbi.nlm.nih.gov:80/entrez/query.fcgi?cmd=Retrieve&db=
  PubMed&list_uids=6275826&dopt=Abstract

- **Valproate metabolites in serum and urine during antiepileptic therapy in children with infantile spasms: abnormal metabolite pattern associated with reversible hepatotoxicity.**
  Author(s): Fisher E, Siemes H, Pund R, Wittfoht W, Nau H.
  Source: Epilepsia. 1992 January-February; 33(1): 165-71.
  http://www.ncbi.nlm.nih.gov:80/entrez/query.fcgi?cmd=Retrieve&db=
  PubMed&list_uids=1733752&dopt=Abstract

- **Vein of Galen malformation and infantile spasms.**
  Author(s): Incorpora G, Pavone P, Platania N, Trifiletti RR, Parano E.
  Source: Journal of Child Neurology. 1999 March; 14(3): 196-8.
  http://www.ncbi.nlm.nih.gov:80/entrez/query.fcgi?cmd=Retrieve&db=
  PubMed&list_uids=10190271&dopt=Abstract

- **Vigabatrin as first line therapy in infantile spasms: review of seven patients.**
  Author(s): Kwong L.
  Source: Journal of Paediatrics and Child Health. 1997 April; 33(2): 121-4.
  http://www.ncbi.nlm.nih.gov:80/entrez/query.fcgi?cmd=Retrieve&db=
  PubMed&list_uids=9145354&dopt=Abstract

- **Vigabatrin as initial therapy for infantile spasms: a European retrospective survey. Sabril IS Investigator and Peer Review Groups.**
  Author(s): Aicardi J, Mumford JP, Dumas C, Wood S.
  Source: Epilepsia. 1996 July; 37(7): 638-42.
  http://www.ncbi.nlm.nih.gov:80/entrez/query.fcgi?cmd=Retrieve&db=
  PubMed&list_uids=8681895&dopt=Abstract

- **Vigabatrin for infantile spasms.**
  Author(s): Mitchell WG, Shah NS.
  Source: Pediatric Neurology. 2002 September; 27(3): 161-4.
  http://www.ncbi.nlm.nih.gov:80/entrez/query.fcgi?cmd=Retrieve&db=
  PubMed&list_uids=12393124&dopt=Abstract

- **Vigabatrin in infantile spasms.**
  Author(s): Chiron C, Dulac O, Luna D, Palacios L, Mondragon S, Beaumont D, Mumford JP.
  Source: Lancet. 1990 February 10; 335(8685): 363-4.
  http://www.ncbi.nlm.nih.gov:80/entrez/query.fcgi?cmd=Retrieve&db=PubMed&list_uids=1967808&dopt=Abstract

- **Vigabatrin in infantile spasms: preliminary result.**
  Author(s): Visudtibhan A, Chiemchanya S, Visudhiphan P, Phusirimongkol S.
  Source: J Med Assoc Thai. 1999 October; 82(10): 1000-5.
  http://www.ncbi.nlm.nih.gov:80/entrez/query.fcgi?cmd=Retrieve&db=PubMed&list_uids=10561962&dopt=Abstract

- **Vigabatrin in infantile spasms--why add on?**
  Author(s): Appleton RE, Montiel-Viesca F.
  Source: Lancet. 1993 April 10; 341(8850): 962.
  http://www.ncbi.nlm.nih.gov:80/entrez/query.fcgi?cmd=Retrieve&db=PubMed&list_uids=8096297&dopt=Abstract

- **Vigabatrin in newly diagnosed infantile spasms.**
  Author(s): Schmitt B, Wohlrab G, Boltshauser E.
  Source: Neuropediatrics. 1994 February; 25(1): 54. Review.
  http://www.ncbi.nlm.nih.gov:80/entrez/query.fcgi?cmd=Retrieve&db=PubMed&list_uids=8208355&dopt=Abstract

- **Vigabatrin in the treatment of infantile spasms in tuberous sclerosis: literature review.**
  Author(s): Hancock E, Osborne JP.
  Source: Journal of Child Neurology. 1999 February; 14(2): 71-4. Review.
  http://www.ncbi.nlm.nih.gov:80/entrez/query.fcgi?cmd=Retrieve&db=PubMed&list_uids=10073425&dopt=Abstract

- **Vigabatrin in the treatment of infantile spasms.**
  Author(s): Koo B.
  Source: Pediatric Neurology. 1999 February; 20(2): 106-10.
  http://www.ncbi.nlm.nih.gov:80/entrez/query.fcgi?cmd=Retrieve&db=PubMed&list_uids=10082337&dopt=Abstract

- **Vigabatrin in the treatment of infantile spasms.**
  Author(s): Vles JS, van der Heyden AM, Ghijs A, Troost J.
  Source: Neuropediatrics. 1993 August; 24(4): 230-1.
  http://www.ncbi.nlm.nih.gov:80/entrez/query.fcgi?cmd=Retrieve&db=
  PubMed&list_uids=8232783&dopt=Abstract

- **Vigabatrin therapy in infantile spasms.**
  Author(s): Kankirawatana P, Raksadawan N, Balangkura K.
  Source: J Med Assoc Thai. 2002 August; 85 Suppl 2: S778-83.
  http://www.ncbi.nlm.nih.gov:80/entrez/query.fcgi?cmd=Retrieve&db=
  PubMed&list_uids=12403260&dopt=Abstract

- **Vigabatrin versus ACTH as first-line treatment for infantile spasms: a randomized, prospective study.**
  Author(s): Vigevano F, Cilio MR.
  Source: Epilepsia. 1997 December; 38(12): 1270-4.
  http://www.ncbi.nlm.nih.gov:80/entrez/query.fcgi?cmd=Retrieve&db=
  PubMed&list_uids=9578521&dopt=Abstract

- **Vitamin B6 and valproic acid in treatment of infantile spasms.**
  Author(s): Ito M, Okuno T, Hattori H, Fujii T, Mikawa H.
  Source: Pediatric Neurology. 1991 March-April; 7(2): 91-6.
  http://www.ncbi.nlm.nih.gov:80/entrez/query.fcgi?cmd=Retrieve&db=
  PubMed&list_uids=1647774&dopt=Abstract

- **West's syndrome (infantile spasms). Clinical description and diagnosis.**
  Author(s): Hrachovy RA.
  Source: Advances in Experimental Medicine and Biology. 2002; 497: 33-50. Review.
  http://www.ncbi.nlm.nih.gov:80/entrez/query.fcgi?cmd=Retrieve&db=
  PubMed&list_uids=11993738&dopt=Abstract

- **X linked mental retardation and infantile spasms in a family: new clinical data and linkage to Xp11.4-Xp22.11.**
  Author(s): Stromme P, Sundet K, Mork C, Cassiman JJ, Fryns JP, Claes S.
  Source: Journal of Medical Genetics. 1999 May; 36(5): 374-8.
  http://www.ncbi.nlm.nih.gov:80/entrez/query.fcgi?cmd=Retrieve&db=
  PubMed&list_uids=10353782&dopt=Abstract

- **X-linked mental retardation and infantile spasms in two brothers.**
  Author(s): Rugtveit J.
  Source: Developmental Medicine and Child Neurology. 1986 August; 28(4): 544-6.
  http://www.ncbi.nlm.nih.gov:80/entrez/query.fcgi?cmd=Retrieve&db=PubMed&list_uids=3758508&dopt=Abstract

Vocabulary Builder

Agenesis: Lack of complete or normal development; congenital absence of an organ or part. [NIH]

Anticonvulsive: An agent that prevents or relieves convulsions. [NIH]

Apnea: Cessation of breathing. [NIH]

Asynchronous: Pacing mode where only one timing interval exists, that between the stimuli. While the duration of this interval may be varied, it is not modified by any sensed event once set. As no sensing occurs, the upper and lower rate intervals are the same as the pacema. [NIH]

Branch: Most commonly used for branches of nerves, but applied also to other structures. [NIH]

Cortisol: A steroid hormone secreted by the adrenal cortex as part of the body's response to stress. [NIH]

Crichton: Twitching of the outer corners of the eyes and the lips indicating syphilitic meningoencephalitis. [NIH]

Deletion: A genetic rearrangement through loss of segments of DNA (chromosomes), bringing sequences, which are normally separated, into close proximity. [NIH]

Discrete: Made up of separate parts or characterized by lesions which do not become blended; not running together; separate. [NIH]

Discrimination: The act of qualitative and/or quantitative differentiation between two or more stimuli. [NIH]

EEG: A graphic recording of the changes in electrical potential associated with the activity of the cerebral cortex made with the electroencephalogram. [NIH]

Endorphin: Opioid peptides derived from beta-lipotropin. Endorphin is the most potent naturally occurring analgesic agent. It is present in pituitary, brain, and peripheral tissues. [NIH]

Epilepsia: An illusional seizure consisting of a rather sudden alteration of the patient's perceptions, indicative of a lesion in the temporal lobes. [NIH]

Epilepticus: Repeated and prolonged epileptic seizures without recovery of consciousness between attacks. [NIH]

Excitability: Property of a cardiac cell whereby, when the cell is depolarized to a critical level (called threshold), the membrane becomes permeable and a regenerative inward current causes an action potential. [NIH]

Excitotoxicity: Excessive exposure to glutamate or related compounds can kill brain neurons, presumably by overstimulating them. [NIH]

Fossa: A cavity, depression, or pit. [NIH]

Genetics: The biological science that deals with the phenomena and mechanisms of heredity. [NIH]

Growth: The progressive development of a living being or part of an organism from its earliest stage to maturity. [NIH]

HLA: A glycoprotein found on the surface of all human leucocytes. The HLA region of chromosome 6 produces four such glycoproteins-A, B, C and D. [NIH]

Homeobox: Distinctive sequence of DNA bases. [NIH]

Insight: The capacity to understand one's own motives, to be aware of one's own psychodynamics, to appreciate the meaning of symbolic behavior. [NIH]

Isoenzyme: Different forms of an enzyme, usually occurring in different tissues. The isoenzymes of a particular enzyme catalyze the same reaction but they differ in some of their properties. [NIH]

Joint: The point of contact between elements of an animal skeleton with the parts that surround and support it. [NIH]

Linkage: The tendency of two or more genes in the same chromosome to remain together from one generation to the next more frequently than expected according to the law of independent assortment. [NIH]

Medial: Lying near the midsaggital plane of the body; opposed to lateral. [NIH]

Modeling: A treatment procedure whereby the therapist presents the target behavior which the learner is to imitate and make part of his repertoire. [NIH]

Monoamine: Enzyme that breaks down dopamine in the astrocytes and microglia. [NIH]

Morphological: Relating to the configuration or the structure of live organs. [NIH]

Networks: Pertaining to a nerve or to the nerves, a meshlike structure of interlocking fibers or strands. [NIH]

Nuclei: A body of specialized protoplasm found in nearly all cells and containing the chromosomes. [NIH]

Papilloma: A benign epithelial neoplasm which may arise from the skin, mucous membranes or glandular ducts. [NIH]

Phenotypes: An organism as observed, i. e. as judged by its visually perceptible characters resulting from the interaction of its genotype with the environment. [NIH]

Schizophrenia: A mental disorder characterized by a special type of disintegration of the personality. [NIH]

Segmental: Describing or pertaining to a structure which is repeated in similar form in successive segments of an organism, or which is undergoing segmentation. [NIH]

Spectroscopic: The recognition of elements through their emission spectra. [NIH]

Temporal: One of the two irregular bones forming part of the lateral surfaces and base of the skull, and containing the organs of hearing. [NIH]

Thalamic: Cell that reaches the lateral nucleus of amygdala. [NIH]

Translocation: The movement of material in solution inside the body of the plant. [NIH]

Ulcer: A localized necrotic lesion of the skin or a mucous surface. [NIH]

CHAPTER 5. PATENTS ON INFANTILE SPASMS

Overview

You can learn about innovations relating to infantile spasms by reading recent patents and patent applications. Patents can be physical innovations (e.g. chemicals, pharmaceuticals, medical equipment) or processes (e.g. treatments or diagnostic procedures). The United States Patent and Trademark Office defines a patent as a grant of a property right to the inventor, issued by the Patent and Trademark Office.[19] Patents, therefore, are intellectual property. For the United States, the term of a new patent is 20 years from the date when the patent application was filed. If the inventor wishes to receive economic benefits, it is likely that the invention will become commercially available within 20 years of the initial filing. It is important to understand, therefore, that an inventor's patent does not indicate that a product or service is or will be commercially available. The patent implies only that the inventor has "the right to exclude others from making, using, offering for sale, or selling" the invention in the United States. While this relates to U.S. patents, similar rules govern foreign patents.

In this chapter, we show you how to locate information on patents and their inventors. If you find a patent that is particularly interesting to you, contact the inventor or the assignee for further information.

---

[19]Adapted from The U. S. Patent and Trademark Office:
http://www.uspto.gov/web/offices/pac/doc/general/whatis.htm.

Patent Applications on Infantile Spasms

As of December 2000, U.S. patent applications are open to public viewing.[20] Applications are patent requests which have yet to be granted (the process to achieve a patent can take several years). The following patent applications have been filed since December 2000 relating to infantile spasms:

- **Use of alprazolam in treatment of disorders of the central nervous system**

  Inventor(s): Wong, Erik H.F.; (Portage, MI)

  Correspondence: Pharmacia Corporation; Global Patent Department; Post Office Box 1027; St. Louis; MO; 63006; US

  Patent Application Number: 20040009971

  Date filed: June 18, 2003

  Abstract: A method of treatment of a central nervous system disorder in a human subject comprises administering to the subject by a suitable route a pharmaceutical composition comprising a therapeutically effective amount of alprazolam, wherein the disorder is selected from amyotrophic lateral sclerosis, Creutzfeldt-Jakob disease, Pick's disease, psychosocial dwarfism, Lennox-Gastaut syndrome, **infantile spasms,** and sexual and gender identity disorders.

  Excerpt(s): This application is a continuation-in-part of application Ser. No. 10/179,706, filed on Jun. 25, 2002. This application also claims priority of U.S. provisional application Serial No. 60/391,275, filed on Jun. 25, 2002.... The present invention relates to use of the benzodiazepine drug alprazolam in treatment of certain disorders of the central nervous system (CNS).... Alprazolam, a member of the 1,4-benzodiazepine class of CNS-active compounds, is an effective anxiolytic and anti-panic agent. The immediate-release alprazolam tablet formulation currently marketed as Xanax.RTM. tablets by Pharmacia Corporation can be prescribed for administration of up to four doses per day for treatment of anxiety and, in some instances, in excess of four doses per day for treatment of panic disorder.

  Web site: http://appft1.uspto.gov/netahtml/PTO/search-bool.html

---

[20] This has been a common practice outside the United States prior to December 2000.

Keeping Current

In order to stay informed about patents and patent applications dealing with infantile spasms, you can access the U.S. Patent Office archive via the Internet at **http://www.uspto.gov/patft/index.html**. You will see two broad options: (1) Issued Patent, and (2) Published Applications. To see a list of issued patents, perform the following steps: Under "Issued Patents," click "Quick Search." Then, type "infantile spasms" (or synonyms) into the "Term 1" box. After clicking on the search button, scroll down to see the various patents which have been granted to date on infantile spasms.

You can also use this procedure to view pending patent applications concerning infantile spasms. Simply go back to the following Web address: **http://www.uspto.gov/patft/index.html**. Select "Quick Search" under "Published Applications." Then proceed with the steps listed above.

CHAPTER 6. BOOKS ON INFANTILE SPASMS

Overview

This chapter provides bibliographic book references relating to infantile spasms. You have many options to locate books on infantile spasms. The simplest method is to go to your local bookseller and inquire about titles that they have in stock or can special order for you. Some parents, however, prefer online sources (e.g. **www.amazon.com** and **www.bn.com**). In addition to online booksellers, excellent sources for book titles on infantile spasms include the Combined Health Information Database and the National Library of Medicine. Once you have found a title that interests you, visit your local public or medical library to see if it is available for loan.

Book Summaries: Online Booksellers

Commercial Internet-based booksellers, such as Amazon.com and Barnes & Noble.com, offer summaries which have been supplied by each title's publisher. Some summaries also include customer reviews. Your local bookseller may have access to in-house and commercial databases that index all published books (e.g. Books in Print®). The following have been recently listed with online booksellers as relating to infantile spasms (sorted alphabetically by title; follow the hyperlink to view more details at Amazon.com):

- **Epilepsy, Infantile Spasms, and Developmental Encephalopathy** by Philip Schwartzkroin (Author), et al; ISBN: 0123668492; http://www.amazon.com/exec/obidos/ASIN/0123668492/icongroupinterna

- **Infantile Spasms** by Joseph R. Lacy; ISBN: 0890040184;
  http://www.amazon.com/exec/obidos/ASIN/0890040184/icongroupin
  terna

- **Infantile Spasms and West Syndrome** by Olivier Dulac (Editor), et al;
  ISBN: 0702017779;
  http://www.amazon.com/exec/obidos/ASIN/0702017779/icongroupin
  terna

- **Infantile Spasms: Diagnosis, Management and Prognosis** by James D.,
  Jr Frost, Richard A. Hrachovy; ISBN: 1402074824;
  http://www.amazon.com/exec/obidos/ASIN/1402074824/icongroupin
  terna

Chapters on Infantile Spasms

Frequently, infantile spasms will be discussed within a book, perhaps within a specific chapter. In order to find chapters that are specifically dealing with infantile spasms, an excellent source of abstracts is the Combined Health Information Database. You will need to limit your search to book chapters and infantile spasms using the "Detailed Search" option. Go directly to the following hyperlink: **http://chid.nih.gov/detail/detail.html**. To find book chapters, use the drop boxes at the bottom of the search page where "You may refine your search by." Select the dates and language you prefer, and the format option "Book Chapter." By making these selections and typing in "infantile spasms" (or synonyms) into the "For these words:" box, you will only receive results on chapters in books.

General Home References

In addition to references for infantile spasms, you may want a general home medical guide that spans all aspects of home healthcare. The following list is a recent sample of such guides (sorted alphabetically by title; hyperlinks provide rankings, information, and reviews at Amazon.com):

- **Adams & Victor's Principles Of Neurology** by Maurice Victor, et al;
  Hardcover - 1692 pages; 7th edition (December 19, 2000), McGraw-Hill
  Professional Publishing; ISBN: 0070674973;
  **http://www.amazon.com/exec/obidos/ASIN/0070674973/icongroupinter
  na**

- **American Academy of Pediatrics Guide to Your Child's Symptoms :
  The Official, Complete Home Reference, Birth Through Adolescence**

by Donald Schiff (Editor), et al; Paperback - 256 pages (January 1997), Villard Books; ISBN: 0375752579; http://www.amazon.com/exec/obidos/ASIN/0375752579/icongroupinterna

- **The Children's Hospital Guide to Your Child's Health and Development** by Alan D. Woolf (Editor), et al; Hardcover - 796 pages, 1st edition (January 15, 2001), Perseus Books; ISBN: 073820241X; http://www.amazon.com/exec/obidos/ASIN/073820241X/icongroupinterna

- **Clinical Neuroanatomy Made Ridiculously Simple (MedMaster Series, 2000 Edition)** by Stephen Goldberg; Paperback: 97 pages; 2nd edition (February 15, 2000), Medmaster; ISBN: 0940780461; http://www.amazon.com/exec/obidos/ASIN/0940780461/icongroupinterna

- **Helping Your Child in the Hospital: A Practical Guide for Parents** by Nancy Keene, Rachel Prentice; Paperback - 176 pages, 3rd edition (April 15, 2002), O'Reilly & Associates; ISBN: 0596500114; http://www.amazon.com/exec/obidos/ASIN/0596500114/icongroupinterna

- **It's Not a Tumor!: The Patient's Guide to Common Neurological Problems** by Robert Wiedemeyer; Paperback: (January 1996), Boxweed Pub; ISBN: 0964740796; http://www.amazon.com/exec/obidos/ASIN/0964740796/icongroupinterna

- **Medical Emergencies & Childhood Illnesses: Includes Your Child's Personal Health Journal (Parent Smart)** by Penny A. Shore, William Sears (Contributor); Paperback - 115 pages (February 2002), Parent Kit Corporation; ISBN: 1896833187; http://www.amazon.com/exec/obidos/ASIN/1896833187/icongroupinterna

- **Neurology for the Non-Neurologist** by William J. Weiner (Editor), Christopher G. Goetz (Editor); Paperback (May 1999), Lippincott, Williams & Wilkins Publishers; ISBN: 0781717078; http://www.amazon.com/exec/obidos/ASIN/0781717078/icongroupinterna

- **Taking Care of Your Child: A Parent's Guide to Complete Medical Care** by Robert H. Pantell, M.D., et al; Paperback - 524 pages, 6th edition (March 5, 2002), Perseus Press; ISBN: 0738206016; http://www.amazon.com/exec/obidos/ASIN/0738206016/icongroupinterna

CHAPTER 7. PERIODICALS AND NEWS ON INFANTILE SPASMS

Overview

Keeping up on the news relating to infantile spasms can be challenging. Subscribing to targeted periodicals can be an effective way to stay abreast of recent developments on infantile spasms. Periodicals include newsletters, magazines, and academic journals.

In this chapter, we suggest a number of news sources and present various periodicals that cover infantile spasms beyond and including those which are published by parent associations mentioned earlier. We will first focus on news services, and then on periodicals. News services, press releases, and newsletters generally use more accessible language, so if you do chose to subscribe to one of the more technical periodicals, make sure that it uses language you can easily follow.

News Services and Press Releases

Well before articles show up in newsletters or the popular press, they may appear in the form of a press release or a public relations announcement. One of the simplest ways of tracking press releases on infantile spasms is to search the news wires. News wires are used by professional journalists, and have existed since the invention of the telegraph. Today, there are several major "wires" that are used by companies, universities, and other organizations to announce new medical breakthroughs. In the following sample of sources, we will briefly describe how to access each service. These services only post recent news intended for public viewing.

PR Newswire

Perhaps the broadest of the wires is PR Newswire Association, Inc. To access this archive, simply go to **http://www.prnewswire.com**. Below the search box, select the option "The last 30 days." In the search box, type "infantile spasms" or synonyms. The search results are shown by order of relevance. When reading these press releases, do not forget that the sponsor of the release may be a company or organization that is trying to sell a particular product or therapy. Their views, therefore, may be biased.

Reuters Health

The Reuters' Medical News and Health eLine databases can be very useful in exploring news archives relating to infantile spasms. While some of the listed articles are free to view, others can be purchased for a nominal fee. To access this archive, go to **http://www.reutershealth.com/en/index.html** and search by "infantile spasms" (or synonyms).

The NIH

Within MEDLINEplus, the NIH has made an agreement with the New York Times Syndicate, the AP News Service, and Reuters to deliver news that can be browsed by the public. Search news releases at **http://www.nlm.nih.gov/medlineplus/alphanews_a.html**. MEDLINEplus allows you to browse across an alphabetical index. Or you can search by date at **http://www.nlm.nih.gov/medlineplus/newsbydate.html**. Often, news items are indexed by MEDLINEplus within their search engine.

Business Wire

Business Wire is similar to PR Newswire. To access this archive, simply go to **http://www.businesswire.com**. You can scan the news by industry category or company name.

Market Wire

Market Wire is more focused on technology than the other wires. To browse the latest press releases by topic, such as alternative medicine, biotechnology, fitness, healthcare, legal, nutrition, and pharmaceuticals, log on to Market Wire's Medical/Health channel at the following hyperlink

http://www.marketwire.com/mw/release_index?channel=MedicalHealth.
Market Wire's home page is http://www.marketwire.com/mw/home. From
here, type "infantile spasms" (or synonyms) into the search box, and click on
"Search News." As this service is technology oriented, you may wish to use
it when searching for press releases covering diagnostic procedures or tests.

Search Engines

Free-to-view news can also be found in the news section of your favorite
search engines (see the health news page at Yahoo:
http://dir.yahoo.com/Health/News_and_Media/, or use this Web site's
general news search page http://news.yahoo.com/. Type in "infantile
spasms" (or synonyms). If you know the name of a company that is relevant
to infantile spasms, you can go to any stock trading Web site (such as
www.etrade.com) and search for the company name there. News items
across various news sources are reported on indicated hyperlinks.

BBC

Covering news from a more European perspective, the British Broadcasting
Corporation (BBC) allows the public free access to their news archive located
at http://www.bbc.co.uk/. Search by "infantile spasms" (or synonyms).

Academic Periodicals covering Infantile Spasms

Academic periodicals can be a highly technical yet valuable source of
information on infantile spasms. We have compiled the following list of
periodicals known to publish articles relating to infantile spasms and which
are currently indexed within the National Library of Medicine's PubMed
database (follow hyperlinks to view more information, summaries, etc., for
each). In addition to these sources, to keep current on articles written on
infantile spasms published by any of the periodicals listed below, you can
simply follow the hyperlink indicated or go to
www.ncbi.nlm.nih.gov/pubmed. Type the periodical's name into the search
box to find the latest studies published.

If you want complete details about the historical contents of a periodical,
visit the Web site: http://www.ncbi.nlm.nih.gov/entrez/jrbrowser.cgi. Here,
type in the name of the journal or its abbreviation, and you will receive an
index of published articles. At http://locatorplus.gov/ you can retrieve more

indexing information on medical periodicals (e.g. the name of the publisher). Select the button "Search LOCATORplus." Then type in the name of the journal and select the advanced search option "Journal Title Search." The following is a sample of periodicals which publish articles on infantile spasms:

- **Acta Neurologica Scandinavica. (Acta Neurol Scand)**
  http://www.ncbi.nlm.nih.gov/entrez/jrbrowser.cgi?field=0&regexp=Acta+Neurologica+Scandinavica&dispmax=20&dispstart=0

- **Acta Paediatrica (Oslo, Norway : 1992). (Acta Paediatr)**
  http://www.ncbi.nlm.nih.gov/entrez/jrbrowser.cgi?field=0&regexp=Acta+Paediatrica+(Oslo,+Norway+:+1992)&dispmax=20&dispstart=0

- **Advances in Experimental Medicine and Biology. (Adv Exp Med Biol)**
  http://www.ncbi.nlm.nih.gov/entrez/jrbrowser.cgi?field=0&regexp=Advances+in+Experimental+Medicine+and+Biology&dispmax=20&dispstart=0

- **Ajnr. American Journal of Neuroradiology. (AJNR Am J Neuroradiol)**
  http://www.ncbi.nlm.nih.gov/entrez/jrbrowser.cgi?field=0&regexp=Ajnr.+American+Journal+of+Neuroradiology&dispmax=20&dispstart=0

- **American Journal of Human Genetics. (Am J Hum Genet)**
  http://www.ncbi.nlm.nih.gov/entrez/jrbrowser.cgi?field=0&regexp=American+Journal+of+Human+Genetics&dispmax=20&dispstart=0

- **American Journal of Kidney Diseases : the Official Journal of the National Kidney Foundation. (Am J Kidney Dis)**
  http://www.ncbi.nlm.nih.gov/entrez/jrbrowser.cgi?field=0&regexp=American+Journal+of+Kidney+Diseases+:+the+Official+Journal+of+the+National+Kidney+Foundation&dispmax=20&dispstart=0

- **Annals of Neurology. (Ann Neurol)**
  http://www.ncbi.nlm.nih.gov/entrez/jrbrowser.cgi?field=0&regexp=Annals+of+Neurology&dispmax=20&dispstart=0

- **Archives of Disease in Childhood. (Arch Dis Child)**
  http://www.ncbi.nlm.nih.gov/entrez/jrbrowser.cgi?field=0&regexp=Archives+of+Disease+in+Childhood&dispmax=20&dispstart=0

- **Archives of Neurology. (Arch Neurol)**
  http://www.ncbi.nlm.nih.gov/entrez/jrbrowser.cgi?field=0&regexp=Archives+of+Neurology&dispmax=20&dispstart=0

- **Bmj (Clinical Research Ed.. (BMJ)**
  http://www.ncbi.nlm.nih.gov/entrez/jrbrowser.cgi?field=0&regexp=Bmj+(Clinical+Research+Ed.+&dispmax=20&dispstart=0

- **Brain & Development. (Brain Dev)**
  http://www.ncbi.nlm.nih.gov/entrez/jrbrowser.cgi?field=0&regexp=Brain+&+Development&dispmax=20&dispstart=0

- **Brain and Cognition. (Brain Cogn)**
  http://www.ncbi.nlm.nih.gov/entrez/jrbrowser.cgi?field=0&regexp=Brain+and+Cognition&dispmax=20&dispstart=0

- **Child's Nervous System : Chns : Official Journal of the International Society for Pediatric Neurosurgery. (Childs Nerv Syst)**
  http://www.ncbi.nlm.nih.gov/entrez/jrbrowser.cgi?field=0&regexp=Child's+Nervous+System+:+Chns+:+Official+Journal+of+the+International+Society+for+Pediatric+Neurosurgery&dispmax=20&dispstart=0

- **Clinical Dysmorphology. (Clin Dysmorphol)**
  http://www.ncbi.nlm.nih.gov/entrez/jrbrowser.cgi?field=0&regexp=Clinical+Dysmorphology&dispmax=20&dispstart=0

- **Clinical Genetics. (Clin Genet)**
  http://www.ncbi.nlm.nih.gov/entrez/jrbrowser.cgi?field=0&regexp=Clinical+Genetics&dispmax=20&dispstart=0

- **Clinical Neurology and Neurosurgery. (Clin Neurol Neurosurg)**
  http://www.ncbi.nlm.nih.gov/entrez/jrbrowser.cgi?field=0&regexp=Clinical+Neurology+and+Neurosurgery&dispmax=20&dispstart=0

- **Clinical Neuropharmacology. (Clin Neuropharmacol)**
  http://www.ncbi.nlm.nih.gov/entrez/jrbrowser.cgi?field=0&regexp=Clinical+Neuropharmacology&dispmax=20&dispstart=0

- **Clinical Neurophysiology : Official Journal of the International Federation of Clinical Neurophysiology. (Clin Neurophysiol)**
  http://www.ncbi.nlm.nih.gov/entrez/jrbrowser.cgi?field=0&regexp=Cli

nical+Neurophysiology+:+Official+Journal+of+the+International+Federa
tion+of+Clinical+Neurophysiology&dispmax=20&dispstart=0

- **Developmental Medicine and Child Neurology. (Dev Med Child Neurol)**
http://www.ncbi.nlm.nih.gov/entrez/jrbrowser.cgi?field=0&regexp=De
velopmental+Medicine+and+Child+Neurology&dispmax=20&dispstart=
0

- **Developmental Neuroscience. (Dev Neurosci)**
http://www.ncbi.nlm.nih.gov/entrez/jrbrowser.cgi?field=0&regexp=De
velopmental+Neuroscience&dispmax=20&dispstart=0

- **Drug Safety : an International Journal of Medical Toxicology and Drug Experience. (Drug Saf)**
http://www.ncbi.nlm.nih.gov/entrez/jrbrowser.cgi?field=0&regexp=Dr
ug+Safety+:+an+International+Journal+of+Medical+Toxicology+and+Dr
ug+Experience&dispmax=20&dispstart=0

- **Electroencephalography and Clinical Neurophysiology. (Electroencephalogr Clin Neurophysiol)**
http://www.ncbi.nlm.nih.gov/entrez/jrbrowser.cgi?field=0&regexp=Ele
ctroencephalography+and+Clinical+Neurophysiology&dispmax=20&dis
pstart=0

- **Epilepsy Research. (Epilepsy Res)**
http://www.ncbi.nlm.nih.gov/entrez/jrbrowser.cgi?field=0&regexp=Ep
ilepsy+Research&dispmax=20&dispstart=0

- **Epileptic Disorders : International Epilepsy Journal with Videotape. (Epileptic Disord)**
http://www.ncbi.nlm.nih.gov/entrez/jrbrowser.cgi?field=0&regexp=Ep
ileptic+Disorders+:+International+Epilepsy+Journal+with+Videotape&di
spmax=20&dispstart=0

- **European Journal of Pediatrics. (Eur J Pediatr)**
http://www.ncbi.nlm.nih.gov/entrez/jrbrowser.cgi?field=0&regexp=Eu
ropean+Journal+of+Pediatrics&dispmax=20&dispstart=0

- **European Neurology. (Eur Neurol)**
http://www.ncbi.nlm.nih.gov/entrez/jrbrowser.cgi?field=0&regexp=Eu

ropean+Neurology&dispmax=20&dispstart=0

- **Expert Opinion on Pharmacotherapy. (Expert Opin Pharmacother)**
  http://www.ncbi.nlm.nih.gov/entrez/jrbrowser.cgi?field=0&regexp=Expert+Opinion+on+Pharmacotherapy&dispmax=20&dispstart=0

- **International Journal of Pediatric Otorhinolaryngology. (Int J Pediatr Otorhinolaryngol)**
  http://www.ncbi.nlm.nih.gov/entrez/jrbrowser.cgi?field=0&regexp=International+Journal+of+Pediatric+Otorhinolaryngology&dispmax=20&dispstart=0

- **Italian Journal of Neurological Sciences. (Ital J Neurol Sci)**
  http://www.ncbi.nlm.nih.gov/entrez/jrbrowser.cgi?field=0&regexp=Italian+Journal+of+Neurological+Sciences&dispmax=20&dispstart=0

- **J Aapos. (J AAPOS)**
  http://www.ncbi.nlm.nih.gov/entrez/jrbrowser.cgi?field=0&regexp=J+Aapos&dispmax=20&dispstart=0

- **Journal of Child Neurology. (J Child Neurol)**
  http://www.ncbi.nlm.nih.gov/entrez/jrbrowser.cgi?field=0&regexp=Journal+of+Child+Neurology&dispmax=20&dispstart=0

- **Journal of Clinical Neurophysiology : Official Publication of the American Electroencephalographic Society. (J Clin Neurophysiol)**
  http://www.ncbi.nlm.nih.gov/entrez/jrbrowser.cgi?field=0&regexp=Journal+of+Clinical+Neurophysiology+:+Official+Publication+of+the+American+Electroencephalographic+Society&dispmax=20&dispstart=0

- **Journal of Human Genetics. (J Hum Genet)**
  http://www.ncbi.nlm.nih.gov/entrez/jrbrowser.cgi?field=0&regexp=Journal+of+Human+Genetics&dispmax=20&dispstart=0

- **Journal of Inherited Metabolic Disease. (J Inherit Metab Dis)**
  http://www.ncbi.nlm.nih.gov/entrez/jrbrowser.cgi?field=0&regexp=Journal+of+Inherited+Metabolic+Disease&dispmax=20&dispstart=0

- **Journal of Medical Genetics. (J Med Genet)**
  http://www.ncbi.nlm.nih.gov/entrez/jrbrowser.cgi?field=0&regexp=Journal+of+Medical+Genetics&dispmax=20&dispstart=0

- **Journal of Neural Transmission (Vienna, Austria : 1996). (J Neural Transm)**
  http://www.ncbi.nlm.nih.gov/entrez/jrbrowser.cgi?field=0&regexp=Journal+of+Neural+Transmission+(Vienna,+Austria+:+1996)&dispmax=20&dispstart=0

- **Journal of Neurology, Neurosurgery, and Psychiatry. (J Neurol Neurosurg Psychiatry)**
  http://www.ncbi.nlm.nih.gov/entrez/jrbrowser.cgi?field=0&regexp=Journal+of+Neurology,+Neurosurgery,+and+Psychiatry&dispmax=20&dispstart=0

- **Journal of Paediatrics and Child Health. (J Paediatr Child Health)**
  http://www.ncbi.nlm.nih.gov/entrez/jrbrowser.cgi?field=0&regexp=Journal+of+Paediatrics+and+Child+Health&dispmax=20&dispstart=0

- **Journal of the Neurological Sciences. (J Neurol Sci)**
  http://www.ncbi.nlm.nih.gov/entrez/jrbrowser.cgi?field=0&regexp=Journal+of+the+Neurological+Sciences&dispmax=20&dispstart=0

- **Neuropathology : Official Journal of the Japanese Society of Neuropathology. (Neuropathology)**
  http://www.ncbi.nlm.nih.gov/entrez/jrbrowser.cgi?field=0&regexp=Neuropathology+:+Official+Journal+of+the+Japanese+Society+of+Neuropathology&dispmax=20&dispstart=0

- **Pediatric Neurology. (Pediatr Neurol)**
  http://www.ncbi.nlm.nih.gov/entrez/jrbrowser.cgi?field=0&regexp=Pediatric+Neurology&dispmax=20&dispstart=0

- **Pediatric Nursing. (Pediatr Nurs)**
  http://www.ncbi.nlm.nih.gov/entrez/jrbrowser.cgi?field=0&regexp=Pediatric+Nursing&dispmax=20&dispstart=0

- **Pediatric Pulmonology. (Pediatr Pulmonol)**
  http://www.ncbi.nlm.nih.gov/entrez/jrbrowser.cgi?field=0&regexp=Pediatric+Pulmonology&dispmax=20&dispstart=0

- **Pediatric Radiology. (Pediatr Radiol)**
  http://www.ncbi.nlm.nih.gov/entrez/jrbrowser.cgi?field=0&regexp=Pe

diatric+Radiology&dispmax=20&dispstart=0

- **Pediatrics International : Official Journal of the Japan Pediatric Society. (Pediatr Int)**
  http://www.ncbi.nlm.nih.gov/entrez/jrbrowser.cgi?field=0&regexp=Pe
  diatrics+International+:+Official+Journal+of+the+Japan+Pediatric+Societ
  y&dispmax=20&dispstart=0

- **Seizure : the Journal of the British Epilepsy Association. (Seizure)**
  http://www.ncbi.nlm.nih.gov/entrez/jrbrowser.cgi?field=0&regexp=Sei
  zure+:+the+Journal+of+the+British+Epilepsy+Association&dispmax=20
  &dispstart=0

- **The Annals of Pharmacotherapy. (Ann Pharmacother)**
  http://www.ncbi.nlm.nih.gov/entrez/jrbrowser.cgi?field=0&regexp=Th
  e+Annals+of+Pharmacotherapy&dispmax=20&dispstart=0

- **The Canadian Journal of Cardiology. (Can J Cardiol)**
  http://www.ncbi.nlm.nih.gov/entrez/jrbrowser.cgi?field=0&regexp=Th
  e+Canadian+Journal+of+Cardiology&dispmax=20&dispstart=0

- **The Canadian Journal of Neurological Sciences. Le Journal Canadien Des Sciences Neurologiques. (Can J Neurol Sci)**
  http://www.ncbi.nlm.nih.gov/entrez/jrbrowser.cgi?field=0&regexp=Th
  e+Canadian+Journal+of+Neurological+Sciences.+Le+Journal+Canadien+
  Des+Sciences+Neurologiques&dispmax=20&dispstart=0

- **The Journal of Neuroscience Nursing : Journal of the American Association of Neuroscience Nurses. (J Neurosci Nurs)**
  http://www.ncbi.nlm.nih.gov/entrez/jrbrowser.cgi?field=0&regexp=Th
  e+Journal+of+Neuroscience+Nursing+:+Journal+of+the+American+Asso
  ciation+of+Neuroscience+Nurses&dispmax=20&dispstart=0

- **The Journal of Pediatrics. (J Pediatr)**
  http://www.ncbi.nlm.nih.gov/entrez/jrbrowser.cgi?field=0&regexp=Th
  e+Journal+of+Pediatrics&dispmax=20&dispstart=0

- **The Nurse Practitioner. (Nurse Pract)**
  http://www.ncbi.nlm.nih.gov/entrez/jrbrowser.cgi?field=0&regexp=Th
  e+Nurse+Practitioner&dispmax=20&dispstart=0

- **The Pediatric Infectious Disease Journal. (Pediatr Infect Dis J)**
  http://www.ncbi.nlm.nih.gov/entrez/jrbrowser.cgi?field=0&regexp=Th
  e+Pediatric+Infectious+Disease+Journal&dispmax=20&dispstart=0

CHAPTER 8. PHYSICIAN GUIDELINES AND DATABASES

Overview

Doctors and medical researchers rely on a number of information sources to help children with infantile spasms. Many will subscribe to journals or newsletters published by their professional associations or refer to specialized textbooks or clinical guides published for the medical profession. In this chapter, we focus on databases and Internet-based guidelines created or written for this professional audience.

NIH Guidelines

For the more common medical conditions, the National Institutes of Health publish guidelines that are frequently consulted by physicians. Publications are typically written by one or more of the various NIH Institutes. For physician guidelines, commonly referred to as "clinical" or "professional" guidelines, you can visit the following Institutes:

- Office of the Director (OD); guidelines consolidated across agencies available at **http://www.nih.gov/health/consumer/conkey.htm**

- National Institute of General Medical Sciences (NIGMS); fact sheets available at **http://www.nigms.nih.gov/news/facts/**

- National Library of Medicine (NLM); extensive encyclopedia (A.D.A.M., Inc.) with guidelines:
  http://www.nlm.nih.gov/medlineplus/healthtopics.html

- National Institute of Neurological Disorders and Stroke (NINDS); neurological disorder information pages available at
  http://www.ninds.nih.gov/health_and_medical/disorder_index.htm

NIH Databases

In addition to the various Institutes of Health that publish professional guidelines, the NIH has designed a number of databases for professionals.[21] Physician-oriented resources provide a wide variety of information related to the biomedical and health sciences, both past and present. The format of these resources varies. Searchable databases, bibliographic citations, full text articles (when available), archival collections, and images are all available. The following are referenced by the National Library of Medicine:[22]

- **Bioethics:** Access to published literature on the ethical, legal and public policy issues surrounding healthcare and biomedical research. This information is provided in conjunction with the Kennedy Institute of Ethics located at Georgetown University, Washington, D.C.: **http://www.nlm.nih.gov/databases/databases_bioethics.html**

- **HIV/AIDS Resources:** Describes various links and databases dedicated to HIV/AIDS research: **http://www.nlm.nih.gov/pubs/factsheets/aidsinfs.html**

- **NLM Online Exhibitions:** Describes "Exhibitions in the History of Medicine": **http://www.nlm.nih.gov/exhibition/exhibition.html**. Additional resources for historical scholarship in medicine: **http://www.nlm.nih.gov/hmd/hmd.html**

- **Biotechnology Information:** Access to public databases. The National Center for Biotechnology Information conducts research in computational biology, develops software tools for analyzing genome data, and disseminates biomedical information for the better understanding of molecular processes affecting human health and disease: **http://www.ncbi.nlm.nih.gov/**

- **Population Information:** The National Library of Medicine provides access to worldwide coverage of population, family planning, and related health issues, including family planning technology and programs, fertility, and population law and policy: **http://www.nlm.nih.gov/databases/databases_population.html**

- **Cancer Information:** Access to caner-oriented databases: **http://www.nlm.nih.gov/databases/databases_cancer.html**

---

[21] Remember, for the general public, the National Library of Medicine recommends the databases referenced in MEDLINE*plus* (**http://medlineplus.gov/** or **http://www.nlm.nih.gov/medlineplus/databases.html**).

[22] See **http://www.nlm.nih.gov/databases/databases.html**.

- **Profiles in Science:** Offering the archival collections of prominent twentieth-century biomedical scientists to the public through modern digital technology: **http://www.profiles.nlm.nih.gov/**

- **Chemical Information:** Provides links to various chemical databases and references: **http://sis.nlm.nih.gov/Chem/ChemMain.html**

- **Clinical Alerts:** Reports the release of findings from the NIH-funded clinical trials where such release could significantly affect morbidity and mortality: **http://www.nlm.nih.gov/databases/alerts/clinical_alerts.html**

- **Space Life Sciences:** Provides links and information to space-based research (including NASA): **http://www.nlm.nih.gov/databases/databases_space.html**

- **MEDLINE:** Bibliographic database covering the fields of medicine, nursing, dentistry, veterinary medicine, the healthcare system, and the pre-clinical sciences: **http://www.nlm.nih.gov/databases/databases_medline.html**

- **Toxicology and Environmental Health Information (TOXNET):** Databases covering toxicology and environmental health: **http://sis.nlm.nih.gov/Tox/ToxMain.html**

- **Visible Human Interface:** Anatomically detailed, three-dimensional representations of normal male and female human bodies: **http://www.nlm.nih.gov/research/visible/visible_human.html**

While all of the above references may be of interest to physicians who study and treat infantile spasms, the following are particularly noteworthy.

The NLM Gateway[23]

The NLM (National Library of Medicine) Gateway is a Web-based system that lets users search simultaneously in multiple retrieval systems at the U.S. National Library of Medicine (NLM). It allows users of NLM services to initiate searches from one Web interface, providing "one-stop searching" for many of NLM's information resources or databases.[24] One target audience for the Gateway is the Internet user who is new to NLM's online resources and does not know what information is available or how best to search for it. This audience may include physicians and other healthcare providers,

---

[23] Adapted from NLM: **http://gateway.nlm.nih.gov/gw/Cmd?Overview.x**.

[24] The NLM Gateway is currently being developed by the Lister Hill National Center for Biomedical Communications (LHNCBC) at the National Library of Medicine (NLM) of the National Institutes of Health (NIH).

researchers, librarians, students, and, increasingly, parents and the public.[25] To use the NLM Gateway, simply go to the search site at **http://gateway.nlm.nih.gov/gw/Cmd**. Type "infantile spasms" (or synonyms) into the search box and click "Search." The results will be presented in a tabular form, indicating the number of references in each database category.

Results Summary

Category	Items Found
Journal Articles	2186
Books / Periodicals / Audio Visual	13
Consumer Health	357
Meeting Abstracts	0
Other Collections	27
Total	2583

HSTAT[26]

HSTAT is a free, Web-based resource that provides access to full-text documents used in healthcare decision-making.[27] HSTAT's audience includes healthcare providers, health service researchers, policy makers, insurance companies, consumers, and the information professionals who serve these groups. HSTAT provides access to a wide variety of publications, including clinical practice guidelines, quick-reference guides for clinicians, consumer health brochures, evidence reports and technology assessments from the Agency for Healthcare Research and Quality (AHRQ), as well as AHRQ's Put Prevention Into Practice.[28] Simply search by "infantile spasms" (or synonyms) at the following Web site: **http://text.nlm.nih.gov**.

---

[25] Other users may find the Gateway useful for an overall search of NLM's information resources. Some searchers may locate what they need immediately, while others will utilize the Gateway as an adjunct tool to other NLM search services such as PubMed® and MEDLINEplus®. The Gateway connects users with multiple NLM retrieval systems while also providing a search interface for its own collections. These collections include various types of information that do not logically belong in PubMed, LOCATORplus, or other established NLM retrieval systems (e.g., meeting announcements and pre-1966 journal citations). The Gateway will provide access to the information found in an increasing number of NLM retrieval systems in several phases.

[26] Adapted from HSTAT: **http://www.nlm.nih.gov/pubs/factsheets/hstat.html**.

[27] The HSTAT URL is **http://hstat.nlm.nih.gov/**.

[28] Other important documents in HSTAT include: the National Institutes of Health (NIH) Consensus Conference Reports and Technology Assessment Reports; the HIV/AIDS Treatment Information Service (ATIS) resource documents; the Substance Abuse and Mental Health Services Administration's Center for Substance Abuse Treatment (SAMHSA/CSAT)

Coffee Break: Tutorials for Biologists[29]

Some parents may wish to have access to a general healthcare site that takes a scientific view of the news and covers recent breakthroughs in biology that may one day assist physicians in developing treatments. To this end, we recommend "Coffee Break," a collection of short reports on recent biological discoveries. Each report incorporates interactive tutorials that demonstrate how bioinformatics tools are used as a part of the research process. Currently, all Coffee Breaks are written by NCBI staff.[30] Each report is about 400 words and is usually based on a discovery reported in one or more articles from recently published, peer-reviewed literature.[31] This site has new articles every few weeks, so it can be considered an online magazine of sorts, and intended for general background information. You can access Coffee Break at **http://www.ncbi.nlm.nih.gov/Coffeebreak/**.

Treatment Improvement Protocols (TIP) and Center for Substance Abuse Prevention (SAMHSA/CSAP) Prevention Enhancement Protocols System (PEPS); the Public Health Service (PHS) Preventive Services Task Force's *Guide to Clinical Preventive Services*; the independent, nonfederal Task Force on Community Services *Guide to Community Preventive Services*; and the Health Technology Advisory Committee (HTAC) of the Minnesota Health Care Commission (MHCC) health technology evaluations.

[29] Adapted from **http://www.ncbi.nlm.nih.gov/Coffeebreak/Archive/FAQ**.html.

[30] The figure that accompanies each article is frequently supplied by an expert external to NCBI, in which case the source of the figure is cited. The result is an interactive tutorial that tells a biological story.

[31] After a brief introduction that sets the work described into a broader context, the report focuses on how a molecular understanding can provide explanations of observed biology and lead to therapies for diseases. Each vignette is accompanied by a figure and hypertext links that lead to a series of pages that interactively show how NCBI tools and resources are used in the research process.

Other Commercial Databases

In addition to resources maintained by official agencies, other databases exist that are commercial ventures addressing medical professionals. Here are some examples that may interest you:

- **CliniWeb International:** Index and table of contents to selected clinical information on the Internet; see **http://www.ohsu.edu/cliniweb/**.

- **Medical World Search:** Searches full text from thousands of selected medical sites on the Internet; see **http://www.mwsearch.com/**.

PART III. APPENDICES

ABOUT PART III

Part III is a collection of appendices on general medical topics relating to infantile spasms and related conditions.

APPENDIX A. RESEARCHING YOUR CHILD'S MEDICATIONS

Overview

There are a number of sources available on new or existing medications which could be prescribed to treat infantile spasms. While a number of hard copy or CD-Rom resources are available to parents and physicians for research purposes, a more flexible method is to use Internet-based databases. In this chapter, we will begin with a general overview of medications. We will then proceed to outline official recommendations on how you should view your child's medications. You may also want to research medications that your child is currently taking for other conditions as they may interact with medications for infantile spasms. Research can give you information on the side effects, interactions, and limitations of prescription drugs used in the treatment of infantile spasms. Broadly speaking, there are two sources of information on approved medications: public sources and private sources. We will emphasize free-to-use public sources.

Your Child's Medications: The Basics[32]

The Agency for Health Care Research and Quality has published extremely useful guidelines on the medication aspects of infantile spasms. Giving your child medication can involve many steps and decisions each day. The AHCRQ recommends that parents take part in treatment decisions. Do not be afraid to ask questions and talk about your concerns. By taking a moment to ask questions, your child may be spared from possible problems. Here are some points to cover each time a new medicine is prescribed:

---

[32] This section is adapted from AHCRQ: **http://www.ahcpr.gov/consumer/ncpiebro.htm**.

- Ask about all parts of your child's treatment, including diet changes, exercise, and medicines.

- Ask about the risks and benefits of each medicine or other treatment your child might receive.

- Ask how often you or your child's doctor will check for side effects from a given medication.

Do not hesitate to tell the doctor about preferences you have for your child's medicines. You may want your child to have a medicine with the fewest side effects, or the fewest doses to take each day. You may care most about cost. Or, you may want the medicine the doctor believes will work the best. Sharing your concerns will help the doctor select the best treatment for your child.

Do not be afraid to "bother" the doctor with your questions about medications for infantile spasms. You can also talk to a nurse or a pharmacist. They can help you better understand your child's treatment plan. Talking over your child's options with someone you trust can help you make better choices. Specifically, ask the doctor the following:

- The name of the medicine and what it is supposed to do.

- How and when to give your child the medicine, how much, and for how long.

- What food, drinks, other medicines, or activities your child should avoid while taking the medicine.

- What side effects your child may experience, and what to do if they occur.

- If there are any refills, and how often.

- About any terms or directions you do not understand.

- What to do if your child misses a dose.

- If there is written information you can take home (most pharmacies have information sheets on prescription medicines; some even offer large-print or Spanish versions).

Do not forget to tell the doctor about all the medicines your child is currently taking (not just those for infantile spasms). This includes prescription medicines and the medicines that you buy over the counter. When talking to the doctor, you may wish to prepare a list of medicines your child is currently taking including why and in what forms. Be sure to include the following information for each:

- Name of medicine

- Reason taken

- Dosage

- Time(s) of day

Also include any over-the-counter medicines, such as:

- Laxatives

- Diet pills

- Vitamins

- Cold medicine

- Aspirin or other pain, headache, or fever medicine

- Cough medicine

- Allergy relief medicine

- Antacids

- Sleeping pills

- Others (include names)

Learning More about Your Child's Medications

Because of historical investments by various organizations and the emergence of the Internet, it has become rather simple to learn about the medications the doctor has recommended for infantile spasms. One such source is the United States Pharmacopeia. In 1820, eleven physicians met in Washington, D.C. to establish the first compendium of standard drugs for the United States. They called this compendium the "U.S. Pharmacopeia (USP)." Today, the USP is a non-profit organization consisting of 800 volunteer scientists, eleven elected officials, and 400 representatives of state associations and colleges of medicine and pharmacy. The USP is located in Rockville, Maryland, and its home page is located at **www.usp.org**. The USP currently provides standards for over 3,700 medications. The resulting USP DI® Advice for the Patient® can be accessed through the National Library of

Medicine of the National Institutes of Health. The database is partially derived from lists of federally approved medications in the Food and Drug Administration's (FDA) Drug Approvals database.[33]

While the FDA database is rather large and difficult to navigate, the Phamacopeia is both user-friendly and free to use. It covers more than 9,000 prescription and over-the-counter medications. To access this database, simply type the following hyperlink into your Web browser: **http://www.nlm.nih.gov/medlineplus/druginformation.html**. To view examples of a given medication (brand names, category, description, preparation, proper use, precautions, side effects, etc.), simply follow the hyperlinks indicated within the United States Pharmacopeia (USP).

Commercial Databases

In addition to the medications listed in the USP above, a number of commercial sites are available by subscription to physicians and their institutions. You may be able to access these sources from your local medical library or your child's doctor's office.

Reuters Health Drug Database

The Reuters Health Drug Database can be searched by keyword at the hyperlink: **http://www.reutershealth.com/frame2/drug.html**.

Mosby's GenRx

Mosby's GenRx database (also available on CD-Rom and book format) covers 45,000 drug products including generics and international brands. It provides information on prescribing and drug interactions. Information can be obtained at the following hyperlink: **http://www.genrx.com/Mosby/PhyGenRx/group.html**.

PDR*health*

The PDR*health* database is a free-to-use, drug information search engine that has been written for the public in layman's terms. It contains FDA-approved

---

[33] Though cumbersome, the FDA database can be freely browsed at the following site: **www.fda.gov/cder/da/da.htm**.

drug information adapted from the Physicians' Desk Reference (PDR) database. PDR*health* can be searched by brand name, generic name, or indication. It features multiple drug interactions reports. Search PDR*health* at **http://www.pdrhealth.com/drug_info/index.html**.

Other Web Sites

A number of additional Web sites discuss drug information. As an example, you may like to look at **www.drugs.com** which reproduces the information in the Pharmacopeia as well as commercial information. You may also want to consider the Web site of the Medical Letter, Inc. which allows users to download articles on various drugs and therapeutics for a nominal fee: **http://www.medletter.com/**.

Researching Orphan Drugs

Orphan drugs are a special class of pharmaceuticals given to patients who are unaffected by existing treatments or with illnesses for which no known drug is effective. Orphan drugs are most commonly prescribed or developed for "rare" medical conditions.[34] According to the FDA, an orphan drug (or biological) may already be approved, or it may still be experimental. A drug becomes an "orphan" when it receives orphan designation from the Office of Orphan Products Development at the FDA.[35] Orphan designation qualifies the sponsor to receive certain benefits from the U.S. Government in exchange for developing the drug. The drug must then undergo the new drug approval process as any other drug would. To date, over 1000 orphan products have been designated, and over 200 have been approved for marketing. Historically, the approval time for orphan products as a group has been considerably shorter than the approval time for other drugs. This is due to the fact that many orphan products receive expedited review because they are developed for serious or life-threatening medical conditions.

---

[34] The U.S. Food and Drug Administration defines a rare disease or condition as "any disease or condition which affects less than 200,000 persons in the United States, or affects more than 200,000 in the United States and for which there is no reasonable expectation that the cost of developing and making available in the United States a drug for such disease or condition will be recovered from sales in the United States of such drug." Adapted from the U.S. Food and Drug Administration: **http://www.fda.gov/opacom/laws/orphandg.htm**.
[35] The following is adapted from the U.S. Food and Drug Administration: **http://www.fda.gov/orphan/faq/index.htm**.

The cost of orphan products is determined by the sponsor of the drug and can vary greatly. Reimbursement rates for drug expenses are set by each insurance company and outlined in your child's policy. Insurance companies will generally reimburse for orphan products that have been approved for marketing, but may not reimburse for products that are considered experimental. Consult the insurance company about specific reimbursement policies. If an orphan product has been approved for marketing, it will be available through the normal pharmaceutical supply channels. If the product has not been approved, the sponsor may make the product available on a compassionate-use basis.[36]

Although the list of orphan drugs is revised on a daily basis, you can quickly research orphan drugs that might be applicable to infantile spasms using the database managed by the National Organization for Rare Disorders, Inc. (NORD), located at **www.raredisease.org**. Simply go to their general search page and select "Orphan Drug Designation Database." On this page (**http://www.rarediseases.org/search/noddsearch.html**), type "infantile spasms" or a synonym into the search box and click "Submit Query." When you see a list of drugs, understand that not all of the drugs may be relevant. Some may have been withdrawn from orphan status. Write down or print out the name of each drug and the relevant contact information. From there, visit the Pharmacopeia Web site and type the name of each orphan drug into the search box at the following Web site: **http://www.nlm.nih.gov/medlineplus/druginformation.html**. Read about each drug in detail and consult your doctor to find out if you might benefit from these medications. You or your physician may need to contact the sponsor or NORD.

NORD conducts "early access programs for investigational new drugs (IND) under the Food and Drug Administration's (FDA's) approval 'Treatment INDs' programs which allow for a limited number of individuals to receive investigational drugs before FDA marketing approval." If the orphan product about which you are seeking information is approved for marketing, information on side effects can be found on the product's label. If the product is not approved, you or the physician should consult the sponsor.

---

[36] For contact information on sponsors of orphan products, contact the Office of Orphan Products Development (**http://www.fda.gov/orphan/**). General inquiries may be routed to the main office: Office of Orphan Products Development (HF-35); Food and Drug Administration, 5600 Fishers Lane, Rockville, MD 20857; Voice: (301) 827-3666 or (800) 300-7469; FAX: (301) 443-4915.

The following is a list of orphan drugs currently listed in the NORD Orphan Drug Designation Database for infantile spasms or related conditions:

- **Vigabation (trade name: Sabril)**
  http://www.rarediseases.org/nord/search/nodd_full?code=1047

- **Ganaxolone**
  http://www.rarediseases.org/nord/search/nodd_full?code=717

Contraindications and Interactions (Hidden Dangers)

Some of the medications mentioned in the previous discussions can be problematic for children with infantile spasms--not because they are used in the treatment process, but because of contraindications, or side effects. Medications with contraindications are those that could react with drugs used to treat infantile spasms or potentially create deleterious side effects in patients with infantile spasms. You should ask the physician about any contraindications, especially as these might apply to other medications that your child may be taking for common ailments.

Drug-drug interactions occur when two or more drugs react with each other. This drug-drug interaction may cause your child to experience an unexpected side effect. Drug interactions may make medications less effective, cause unexpected side effects, or increase the action of a particular drug. Some drug interactions can even be harmful to your child.

Be sure to read the label every time you give your child a nonprescription or prescription drug, and take the time to learn about drug interactions. These precautions may be critical to your child's health. You can reduce the risk of potentially harmful drug interactions and side effects with a little bit of knowledge and common sense.

Drug labels contain important information about ingredients, uses, warnings, and directions which you should take the time to read and understand. Labels also include warnings about possible drug interactions. Further, drug labels may change as new information becomes avaiable. This is why it's especially important to read the label every time you give your child a medication. When the doctor prescribes a new drug, discuss all over-the-counter and prescription medications, dietary supplements, vitamins, botanicals, minerals and herbals your child takes. Ask your pharmacist for the package insert for each drug prescribed. The package insert provides more information about potential drug interactions.

A Final Warning

At some point, you may hear of alternative medications from friends, relatives, or in the news media. Advertisements may suggest that certain alternative drugs can produce positive results for infantile spasms. Exercise caution--some of these drugs may have fraudulent claims, and others may actually hurt your child. The Food and Drug Administration (FDA) is the official U.S. agency charged with discovering which medications are likely to improve the health of patients with infantile spasms. The FDA warns to watch out for[37]:

- Secret formulas (real scientists share what they know)
- Amazing breakthroughs or miracle cures (real breakthroughs don't happen very often; when they do, real scientists do not call them amazing or miracles)
- Quick, painless, or guaranteed cures
- If it sounds too good to be true, it probably isn't true.

If you have any questions about any kind of medical treatment, the FDA may have an office near you. Look for their number in the blue pages of the phone book. You can also contact the FDA through its toll-free number, 1-888-INFO-FDA (1-888-463-6332), or on the World Wide Web at **www.fda.gov**.

General References

In addition to the resources provided earlier in this chapter, the following general references describe medications (sorted alphabetically by title; hyperlinks provide rankings, information and reviews at Amazon.com):

- **Current Therapy in Neurologic Disease** by Richard T. Johnson, et al; Hardcover - 457 pages, 6th edition (January 15, 2002), Mosby-Year Book; ISBN: 0323014720; **http://www.amazon.com/exec/obidos/ASIN/0323014720/icongroupinter na**

- **Emerging Pharmacological Tools in Clinical Neurology** by MedPanel Inc. (Author); Digital - 66 pages, MarketResearch.com; ISBN: B00005RBN8; **http://www.amazon.com/exec/obidos/ASIN/B00005RBN8/icongroupint erna**

---

[37] This section has been adapted from **http://www.fda.gov/opacom/lowlit/medfraud.html**.

- **Goodman & Gilman's The Pharmacological Basis of Therapeutics by** Joel G. Hardman (Editor), Lee E. Limbird; Hardcover - 1825 pages, 10th edition (August 13, 2001), McGraw-Hill Professional Publishing; ISBN: 0071354697;
  http://www.amazon.com/exec/obidos/ASIN/0071354697/icongroupinterna

- **Neurology and General Medicine** by Michael J. Aminoff (Editor), Hardcover - 992 pages, 3rd edition (March 15, 2001), Churchill Livingstone; ISBN: 0443065713;
  http://www.amazon.com/exec/obidos/ASIN/0443065713/icongroupinterna

- **Neurology and Medicine** by Hughes Perkins; Hardcover - 415 pages, 1st edition (December 15, 1999), B. M. J. Books; ISBN: 0727912240;
  http://www.amazon.com/exec/obidos/ASIN/0727912240/icongroupinterna

- **Pharmacological Management of Neurological and Psychiatric Disorders** by S. J. Enna (Editor), et al; Hardcover - 736 pages, 1st edition, McGraw-Hill Professional Publishing; ISBN: 0070217645;
  http://www.amazon.com/exec/obidos/ASIN/0070217645/icongroupinterna

Vocabulary Builder

The following vocabulary builder gives definitions of words used in this chapter that have not been defined in previous chapters:

Compassionate: A process for providing experimental drugs to very sick patients who have no treatment options. [NIH]

Contraindications: Any factor or sign that it is unwise to pursue a certain kind of action or treatment, e. g. giving a general anesthetic to a person with pneumonia. [NIH]

Therapeutics: The branch of medicine which is concerned with the treatment of diseases, palliative or curative. [NIH]

APPENDIX B. RESEARCHING ALTERNATIVE MEDICINE

Overview

Complementary and alternative medicine (CAM) is one of the most contentious aspects of modern medical practice. You may have heard of these treatments on the radio or on television. Maybe you have seen articles written about these treatments in magazines, newspapers, or books. Perhaps your child's doctor or your friends have mentioned alternatives.

In this chapter, we will begin by giving you a broad perspective on complementary and alternative therapies. Next, we will introduce you to official information sources on CAM relating to infantile spasms. Finally, at the conclusion of this chapter, we will provide a list of readings on infantile spasms from various authors. We will begin, however, with the National Center for Complementary and Alternative Medicine's (NCCAM) overview of complementary and alternative medicine.

What Is CAM?[38]

Complementary and alternative medicine (CAM) covers a broad range of healing philosophies, approaches, and therapies. Generally, it is defined as those treatments and healthcare practices which are not taught in medical schools, used in hospitals, or reimbursed by medical insurance companies. Many CAM therapies are termed "holistic," which generally means that the healthcare practitioner considers the whole person, including physical, mental, emotional, and spiritual health. Some of these therapies are also known as "preventive," which means that the practitioner educates and

---

[38] Adapted from the NCCAM: **http://nccam.nih.gov/health/whatiscam/#4**.

treats the person to prevent health problems from arising, rather than treating symptoms after problems have occurred.

People use CAM treatments and therapies in a variety of ways. Therapies are used alone (often referred to as alternative), in combination with other alternative therapies, or in addition to conventional treatment (sometimes referred to as complementary). Complementary and alternative medicine, or "integrative medicine," includes a broad range of healing philosophies, approaches, and therapies. Some approaches are consistent with physiological principles of Western medicine, while others constitute healing systems with non-Western origins. While some therapies are far outside the realm of accepted Western medical theory and practice, others are becoming established in mainstream medicine.

Complementary and alternative therapies are used in an effort to prevent illness, reduce stress, prevent or reduce side effects and symptoms, or control or cure disease. Some commonly used methods of complementary or alternative therapy include mind/body control interventions such as visualization and relaxation, manual healing including acupressure and massage, homeopathy, vitamins or herbal products, and acupuncture.

What Are the Domains of Alternative Medicine?[39]

The list of CAM practices changes continually. The reason being is that these new practices and therapies are often proved to be safe and effective, and therefore become generally accepted as "mainstream" healthcare practices. Today, CAM practices may be grouped within five major domains: (1) alternative medical systems, (2) mind-body interventions, (3) biologically-based treatments, (4) manipulative and body-based methods, and (5) energy therapies. The individual systems and treatments comprising these categories are too numerous to list in this sourcebook. Thus, only limited examples are provided within each.

Alternative Medical Systems

Alternative medical systems involve complete systems of theory and practice that have evolved independent of, and often prior to, conventional biomedical approaches. Many are traditional systems of medicine that are

---

[39] Adapted from the NCCAM: **http://nccam.nih.gov/health/whatiscam/#4**.

practiced by individual cultures throughout the world, including a number of venerable Asian approaches.

Traditional oriental medicine emphasizes the balance or disturbances of qi (pronounced chi) or vital energy in health and illness, respectively. Traditional oriental medicine consists of a group of techniques and methods including acupuncture, herbal medicine, oriental massage, and qi gong (a form of energy therapy). Acupuncture involves stimulating specific anatomic points in the body for therapeutic purposes, usually by puncturing the skin with a thin needle.

Ayurveda is India's traditional system of medicine. Ayurvedic medicine (meaning "science of life") is a comprehensive system of medicine that places equal emphasis on body, mind, and spirit. Ayurveda strives to restore the innate harmony of the individual. Some of the primary Ayurvedic treatments include diet, exercise, meditation, herbs, massage, exposure to sunlight, and controlled breathing.

Other traditional healing systems have been developed by the world's indigenous populations. These populations include Native American, Aboriginal, African, Middle Eastern, Tibetan, and Central and South American cultures. Homeopathy and naturopathy are also examples of complete alternative medicine systems.

Homeopathic medicine is an unconventional Western system that is based on the principle that "like cures like," i.e., that the same substance that in large doses produces the symptoms of an illness, in very minute doses cures it. Homeopathic health practitioners believe that the more dilute the remedy, the greater its potency. Therefore, they use small doses of specially prepared plant extracts and minerals to stimulate the body's defense mechanisms and healing processes in order to treat illness.

Naturopathic medicine is based on the theory that a medical condition is the manifestation of alterations in the processes by which the body naturally heals itself and emphasizes health restoration rather than treatment for the condition itself. Naturopathic physicians employ an array of healing practices, including the following: diet and clinical nutrition, homeopathy, acupuncture, herbal medicine, hydrotherapy (the use of water in a range of temperatures and methods of applications), spinal and soft-tissue manipulation, physical therapies (such as those involving electrical currents, ultrasound, and light), therapeutic counseling, and pharmacology.

Mind-Body Interventions

Mind-body interventions employ a variety of techniques designed to facilitate the mind's capacity to affect bodily function and symptoms. Only a select group of mind-body interventions having well-documented theoretical foundations are considered CAM. For example, patient education and cognitive-behavioral approaches are now considered "mainstream." On the other hand, complementary and alternative medicine includes meditation, certain uses of hypnosis, dance, music, and art therapy, as well as prayer and mental healing.

Biological-Based Therapies

This category of CAM includes natural and biological-based practices, interventions, and products, many of which overlap with conventional medicine's use of dietary supplements. This category includes herbal, special dietary, orthomolecular, and individual biological therapies.

Herbal therapy employs an individual herb or a mixture of herbs for healing purposes. An herb is a plant or plant part that produces and contains chemical substances that act upon the body. Special diet therapies, such as those proposed by Drs. Atkins, Ornish, Pritikin, and Weil, are believed to prevent and/or control illness as well as promote health. Orthomolecular therapies aim to treat medical conditions with varying concentrations of chemicals such as magnesium, melatonin, and mega-doses of vitamins. Biological therapies include, for example, the use of laetrile and shark cartilage to treat cancer and the use of bee pollen to treat autoimmune and inflammatory conditions.

Manipulative and Body-Based Methods

This category includes methods that are based on manipulation and/or movement of the body. For example, chiropractors focus on the relationship between structure and function, primarily pertaining to the spine, and how that relationship affects the preservation and restoration of health. Chiropractors use manipulative therapy as an integral treatment tool.

In contrast, osteopaths place particular emphasis on the musculoskeletal system and practice osteopathic manipulation. Osteopaths believe that all of the body's systems work together and that disturbances in one system may have an impact upon function elsewhere in the body. Massage therapists manipulate the soft tissues of the body to normalize those tissues.

Energy Therapies

Energy therapies focus on energy fields originating within the body (biofields) or those from other sources (electromagnetic fields). Biofield therapies are intended to affect energy fields (the existence of which is not yet experimentally proven) that surround and penetrate the human body. Some forms of energy therapy manipulate biofields by applying pressure and/or manipulating the body by placing the hands in or through these fields. Examples include Qi gong, Reiki and Therapeutic Touch.

Qi gong is a component of traditional oriental medicine that combines movement, meditation, and regulation of breathing to enhance the flow of vital energy (qi) in the body, improve blood circulation, and enhance immune function. Reiki, the Japanese word representing Universal Life Energy, is based on the belief that, by channeling spiritual energy through the practitioner, the spirit is healed and, in turn, heals the physical body. Therapeutic Touch is derived from the ancient technique of "laying-on of hands." It is based on the premises that the therapist's healing force affects recovery and that healing is promoted when the body's energies are in balance. By passing their hands over the patient, these healers identify energy imbalances.

Bioelectromagnetic-based therapies involve the unconventional use of electromagnetic fields to treat illnesses or manage pain. These therapies are often used to treat asthma, cancer, and migraine headaches. Types of electromagnetic fields which are manipulated in these therapies include pulsed fields, magnetic fields, and alternating current or direct current fields.

Can Alternatives Affect My Child's Treatment?

A critical issue in pursuing complementary alternatives mentioned thus far is the risk that these might have undesirable interactions with your child's medical treatment. It becomes all the more important to speak with the doctor who can offer advice on the use of alternatives. Official sources confirm this view. Though written for women, we find that the National

Women's Health Information Center's advice on pursuing alternative medicine is appropriate for everyone.[40]

Is It Okay to Want Both Traditional and Alternative or Complementary Medicine?

Should you wish to explore non-traditional types of treatment, be sure to discuss all issues concerning treatments and therapies with your child's healthcare provider, whether a physician or practitioner of complementary and alternative medicine. Competent healthcare management requires that the practitioner know of all conventional and alternative therapies that your child is taking.

The decision to use complementary and alternative treatments is an important one. Consider before selecting an alternative therapy, the safety and effectiveness of the therapy or treatment, the expertise and qualifications of the healthcare practitioner, and the quality of delivery. These topics should be considered when selecting any practitioner or therapy.

National Center for Complementary and Alternative Medicine

The National Center for Complementary and Alternative Medicine (NCCAM) of the National Institutes of Health (**http://nccam.nih.gov**) has created a link to the National Library of Medicine's databases to allow parents to search for articles that specifically relate to infantile spasms and complementary medicine. To search the database, go to **www.nlm.nih.gov/nccam/camonpubmed.html**. Select "CAM on PubMed." Enter "infantile spasms" (or synonyms) into the search box. Click "Go." The following references provide information on particular aspects of complementary and alternative medicine (CAM) that are related to infantile spasms:

- **A risk-benefit assessment of treatments for infantile spasms.**
  Author(s): Nabbout R.
  Source: Drug Safety : an International Journal of Medical Toxicology and Drug Experience. 2001; 24(11): 813-28. Review.
  http://www.ncbi.nlm.nih.gov:80/entrez/query.fcgi?cmd=Retrieve&db=PubMed&list_uids=11665869&dopt=Abstract

---

[40] Adapted from **http://www.4woman.gov/faq/alternative.htm**.

- **ACTH therapy for infantile spasms: a combination therapy with high-dose pyridoxal phosphate and low-dose ACTH.**
  Author(s): Takuma Y.
  Source: Epilepsia. 1998; 39 Suppl 5: 42-5.
  http://www.ncbi.nlm.nih.gov:80/entrez/query.fcgi?cmd=Retrieve&db=PubMed&list_uids=9737444&dopt=Abstract

- **Alternative epilepsy therapies: the ketogenic diet, immunoglobulins, and steroids.**
  Author(s): Prasad AN, Stafstrom CF, Holmes GL.
  Source: Epilepsia. 1996; 37 Suppl 1: S81-95. Review.
  http://www.ncbi.nlm.nih.gov:80/entrez/query.fcgi?cmd=Retrieve&db=PubMed&list_uids=8647056&dopt=Abstract

- **Auditory brainstem response: a comparative study of ipsilateral versus contralateral recording in neurological disorders of children.**
  Author(s): Furune S, Watanabe K, Negoro T, Yamamoto N, Aso K, Takaesu E.
  Source: Brain & Development. 1985; 7(5): 463-9.
  http://www.ncbi.nlm.nih.gov:80/entrez/query.fcgi?cmd=Retrieve&db=PubMed&list_uids=4083382&dopt=Abstract

- **Cerebrospinal fluid somatostatin in West syndrome: changes in response to combined treatment with high-dose pyridoxal phosphate and low-dose corticotropin.**
  Author(s): Hirai K, Seki T, Takuma Y.
  Source: Neuropeptides. 1998 December; 32(6): 581-6.
  http://www.ncbi.nlm.nih.gov:80/entrez/query.fcgi?cmd=Retrieve&db=PubMed&list_uids=9920458&dopt=Abstract

- **Combination therapy of infantile spasms with high-dose pyridoxal phosphate and low-dose corticotropin.**
  Author(s): Takuma Y, Seki T.
  Source: Journal of Child Neurology. 1996 January; 11(1): 35-40.
  http://www.ncbi.nlm.nih.gov:80/entrez/query.fcgi?cmd=Retrieve&db=PubMed&list_uids=8745383&dopt=Abstract

- **Combination treatment of high-dose pyridoxal phosphate and low-dose ACTH in children with West syndrome and related disorders.**
  Author(s): Seki T.

Source: Jpn J Psychiatry Neurol. 1990 June; 44(2): 219-37.
http://www.ncbi.nlm.nih.gov:80/entrez/query.fcgi?cmd=Retrieve&db=
PubMed&list_uids=1701836&dopt=Abstract

- **Contact a family: a parent's story.**
  Author(s): Samuel E.
  Source: Paediatric Nursing. 1995 July; 7(6): 9-10.
  http://www.ncbi.nlm.nih.gov:80/entrez/query.fcgi?cmd=Retrieve&db=
  PubMed&list_uids=7627592&dopt=Abstract

- **Diet enriched with omega-3 fatty acids alleviates convulsion symptoms
  in epilepsy patients.**
  Author(s): Schlanger S, Shinitzky M, Yam D.
  Source: Epilepsia. 2002 January; 43(1): 103-4.
  http://www.ncbi.nlm.nih.gov:80/entrez/query.fcgi?cmd=Retrieve&db=
  PubMed&list_uids=11879394&dopt=Abstract

- **Efficacy of the ketogenic diet for infantile spasms.**
  Author(s): Kossoff EH, Pyzik PL, McGrogan JR, Vining EP, Freeman JM.
  Source: Pediatrics. 2002 May; 109(5): 780-3.
  http://www.ncbi.nlm.nih.gov:80/entrez/query.fcgi?cmd=Retrieve&db=
  PubMed&list_uids=11986436&dopt=Abstract

- **Epilepsy in children.**
  Author(s): Arnold ST, Dodson WE.
  Source: Baillieres Clin Neurol. 1996 December; 5(4): 783-802. Review.
  http://www.ncbi.nlm.nih.gov:80/entrez/query.fcgi?cmd=Retrieve&db=
  PubMed&list_uids=9068881&dopt=Abstract

- **Experience with the ketogenic diet in infants.**
  Author(s): Nordli DR Jr, Kuroda MM, Carroll J, Koenigsberger DY,
  Hirsch LJ, Bruner HJ, Seidel WT, De Vivo DC.
  Source: Pediatrics. 2001 July; 108(1): 129-33.
  http://www.ncbi.nlm.nih.gov:80/entrez/query.fcgi?cmd=Retrieve&db=
  PubMed&list_uids=11433065&dopt=Abstract

- **High dose B6 treatment in infantile spasms.**
  Author(s): Blennow G, Starck L.
  Source: Neuropediatrics. 1986 February; 17(1): 7-10.
  http://www.ncbi.nlm.nih.gov:80/entrez/query.fcgi?cmd=Retrieve&db=
  PubMed&list_uids=3960285&dopt=Abstract

- **High-dose vitamin B(6) treatment in West syndrome.**
  Author(s): Toribe Y.
  Source: Brain & Development. 2001 November; 23(7): 654-7. Review.
  http://www.ncbi.nlm.nih.gov:80/entrez/query.fcgi?cmd=Retrieve&db=
  PubMed&list_uids=11701272&dopt=Abstract

- **Improvement of modern treatment and outcome in childhood epilepsy in Asia.**
  Author(s): Chi CS.
  Source: Acta Paediatr Jpn. 1989 June; 31(3): 278-85. Review.
  http://www.ncbi.nlm.nih.gov:80/entrez/query.fcgi?cmd=Retrieve&db=
  PubMed&list_uids=2552743&dopt=Abstract

- **Infantile spasms and Lennox-Gastaut syndrome.**
  Author(s): Trevathan E.
  Source: Journal of Child Neurology. 2002 February; 17 Suppl 2: 2S9-2S22.
  Review. Erratum In: J Child Neurol. 2003 May; 18(5): 374.
  http://www.ncbi.nlm.nih.gov:80/entrez/query.fcgi?cmd=Retrieve&db=
  PubMed&list_uids=11952036&dopt=Abstract

- **Medical treatment of patients with infantile spasms.**
  Author(s): Mikati MA, Lepejian GA, Holmes GL.
  Source: Clinical Neuropharmacology. 2002 March-April; 25(2): 61-70.
  Review.
  http://www.ncbi.nlm.nih.gov:80/entrez/query.fcgi?cmd=Retrieve&db=
  PubMed&list_uids=11981230&dopt=Abstract

- **Newer antiepileptic drugs and non surgical approaches in epilepsy.**
  Author(s): Singhi PD.
  Source: Indian J Pediatr. 2000 January; 67(1 Suppl): S92-8. Review.
  http://www.ncbi.nlm.nih.gov:80/entrez/query.fcgi?cmd=Retrieve&db=
  PubMed&list_uids=11129899&dopt=Abstract

- **Newer GABAergic agents for pharmacotherapy of infantile spasms.**
  Author(s): Reddy DS.
  Source: Drugs Today (Barc). 2002 October; 38(10): 657-75. Review.
  http://www.ncbi.nlm.nih.gov:80/entrez/query.fcgi?cmd=Retrieve&db=
  PubMed&list_uids=12582452&dopt=Abstract

- **Reduction of epileptic seizures through EEG biofeedback training.**
  Author(s): Seifert AR, Lubar JF.

Source: Biological Psychology. 1975 November; 3(3): 157-84.
http://www.ncbi.nlm.nih.gov:80/entrez/query.fcgi?cmd=Retrieve&db=
PubMed&list_uids=812560&dopt=Abstract

- **The role of carnitine supplementation during valproic acid therapy.**
  Author(s): Raskind JY, El-Chaar GM.
  Source: The Annals of Pharmacotherapy. 2000 May; 34(5): 630-8. Review.
  http://www.ncbi.nlm.nih.gov:80/entrez/query.fcgi?cmd=Retrieve&db=
  PubMed&list_uids=10852092&dopt=Abstract

- **The use of sulthiame- in myoclonic epilepsy of childhood and
  adolescence.**
  Author(s): Lerman P, Nussbaum E.
  Source: Acta Neurologica Scandinavica. Supplementum. 1975; 60: 7-12.
  http://www.ncbi.nlm.nih.gov:80/entrez/query.fcgi?cmd=Retrieve&db=
  PubMed&list_uids=242184&dopt=Abstract

- **Treatment of infantile spasms with high-dosage vitamin B6.**
  Author(s): Pietz J, Benninger C, Schafer H, Sontheimer D, Mittermaier G,
  Rating D.
  Source: Epilepsia. 1993 July-August; 34(4): 757-63.
  http://www.ncbi.nlm.nih.gov:80/entrez/query.fcgi?cmd=Retrieve&db=
  PubMed&list_uids=8330589&dopt=Abstract

- **Treatment of the West syndrome with high-dose pyridoxal phosphate.**
  Author(s): Ohtsuka Y, Matsuda M, Ogino T, Kobayashi K, Ohtahara S.
  Source: Brain & Development. 1987; 9(4): 418-21.
  http://www.ncbi.nlm.nih.gov:80/entrez/query.fcgi?cmd=Retrieve&db=
  PubMed&list_uids=3434717&dopt=Abstract

Additional Web Resources

A number of additional Web sites offer encyclopedic information covering
CAM and related topics. The following is a representative sample:

- Alternative Medicine Foundation, Inc.: **http://www.herbmed.org/**
- AOL: **http://search.aol.com/cat.adp?id=169&layer=&from=subcats**
- Chinese Medicine: **http://www.newcenturynutrition.com/**
- Family Village: **http://www.familyvillage.wisc.edu/med_altn.htm**
- Google: **http://directory.google.com/Top/Health/Alternative/**

- Open Directory Project: **http://dmoz.org/Health/Alternative/**
- TPN.com: **http://www.tnp.com/**
- Yahoo.com: **http://dir.yahoo.com/Health/Alternative_Medicine/**
- WebMD®Health: **http://my.webmd.com/drugs_and_herbs**
- WholeHealthMD.com:
  http://www.wholehealthmd.com/reflib/0,1529,,00.html

The following is a specific Web list relating to Infantile Spasms; please note that any particular subject below may indicate either a therapeutic use, or a contraindication (potential danger), and does not reflect an official recommendation:

- **Herbs and Supplements**

  Valproic Acid
  Source: Healthnotes, Inc.; www.healthnotes.com

General References

A good place to find general background information on CAM is the National Library of Medicine. It has prepared within the MEDLINEplus system an information topic page dedicated to complementary and alternative medicine. To access this page, go to the MEDLINEplus site at: **www.nlm.nih.gov/medlineplus/alternativemedicine.html.** This Web site provides a general overview of various topics and can lead to a number of general sources. The following additional references describe, in broad terms, alternative and complementary medicine (sorted alphabetically by title; hyperlinks provide rankings, information, and reviews at Amazon.com):

- **Alternative and Complementary Treatment in Neurologic Illness** by Michael I. Weintraub (Editor); Paperback - 288 pages (March 23, 2001), Churchill Livingstone; ISBN: 0443065586;
  http://www.amazon.com/exec/obidos/ASIN/0443065586/icongroupinterna

- **Healthy Child, Whole Child: Integrating the Best of Conventional and Alternative Medicine to Keep Your Kids Healthy** by Stuart H. Ditchek, M.D. and Russell H. Greenfield; Paperback - 464 pages (June 2002), Harper Resource; ISBN: 0062737465;

http://www.amazon.com/exec/obidos/ASIN/0062737465/icongroupinterna

- **Radical Healing: Integrating the World's Great Therapeutic Traditions to Create a New Transformative Medicine** by Rudolph Ballentine, M.D., Linda Funk (Illustrator); Paperback - 612 pages; Reprint edition (March 14, 2000), Three Rivers Press; ISBN: 0609804847; http://www.amazon.com/exec/obidos/ASIN/0609804847/icongroupinterna

- **The Review of Natural Products** by Facts and Comparisons (Editor); Cd-Rom edition (January 2002), Facts & Comparisons; ISBN: 1574391453; http://www.amazon.com/exec/obidos/ASIN/1574391453/icongroupinterna

For additional information on complementary and alternative medicine, ask your child's doctor or write to:

> **National Center for Complementary and Alternative Medicine Clearinghouse**
> National Institutes of Health
> P. O. Box 8218
> Silver Spring, MD 20907-8218

Vocabulary Builder

The following vocabulary builder gives definitions of words used in this chapter that have not been defined in previous chapters:

Harmony: Attribute of a product which gives rise to an overall pleasant sensation. This sensation is produced by the perception of the product components as olfactory, gustatory, tactile and kinaesthetic stimuli because they are present in suitable concentration ratios. [NIH]

Vivo: Outside of or removed from the body of a living organism. [NIH]

Appendix C. Researching Nutrition

Overview

Since the time of Hippocrates, doctors have understood the importance of diet and nutrition to health and well-being. Since then, they have accumulated an impressive archive of studies and knowledge dedicated to this subject. Based on their experience, doctors and healthcare providers may recommend particular dietary supplements for infantile spasms. Any dietary recommendation is based on age, body mass, gender, lifestyle, eating habits, food preferences, and health condition. It is therefore likely that different patients with infantile spasms may be given different recommendations. Some recommendations may be directly related to infantile spasms, while others may be more related to general health.

In this chapter we will begin by briefly reviewing the essentials of diet and nutrition that will broadly frame more detailed discussions of infantile spasms. We will then show you how to find studies dedicated specifically to nutrition and infantile spasms.

Food and Nutrition: General Principles

What Are Essential Foods?

Food is generally viewed by official sources as consisting of six basic elements: (1) fluids, (2) carbohydrates, (3) protein, (4) fats, (5) vitamins, and (6) minerals. Consuming a combination of these elements is considered to be a healthy diet:

- **Fluids** are essential to human life as 80-percent of the body is composed of water. Water is lost via urination, sweating, diarrhea, vomiting, diuretics (drugs that increase urination), caffeine, and physical exertion.

- **Carbohydrates** are the main source for human energy (thermoregulation) and the bulk of typical diets. They are mostly classified as being either simple or complex. Simple carbohydrates include sugars which are often consumed in the form of cookies, candies, or cakes. Complex carbohydrates consist of starches and dietary fibers. Starches are consumed in the form of pastas, breads, potatoes, rice, and other foods. Soluble fibers can be eaten in the form of certain vegetables, fruits, oats, and legumes. Insoluble fibers include brown rice, whole grains, certain fruits, wheat bran and legumes.

- **Proteins** are eaten to build and repair human tissues. Some foods that are high in protein are also high in fat and calories. Food sources for protein include nuts, meat, fish, cheese, and other dairy products.

- **Fats** are consumed for both energy and the absorption of certain vitamins. There are many types of fats, with many general publications recommending the intake of unsaturated fats or those low in cholesterol.

Vitamins and minerals are fundamental to human health, growth, and, in some cases, disease prevention. Most are consumed in your child's diet (exceptions being vitamins K and D which are produced by intestinal bacteria and sunlight on the skin, respectively). Each vitamin and mineral plays a different role in health. The following outlines essential vitamins:

- **Vitamin A** is important to the health of eyes, hair, bones, and skin; sources of vitamin A include foods such as eggs, carrots, and cantaloupe.

- **Vitamin B^1**, also known as thiamine, is important for the nervous system and energy production; food sources for thiamine include meat, peas, fortified cereals, bread, and whole grains.

- **Vitamin B^2**, also known as riboflavin, is important for the nervous system and muscles, but is also involved in the release of proteins from nutrients; food sources for riboflavin include dairy products, leafy vegetables, meat, and eggs.

- **Vitamin B^3**, also known as niacin, is important for healthy skin and helps the body use energy; food sources for niacin include peas, peanuts, fish, and whole grains

- **Vitamin B^6**, also known as pyridoxine, is important for the regulation of cells in the nervous system and is vital for blood formation; food sources for pyridoxine include bananas, whole grains, meat, and fish.

- **Vitamin B^{12}** is vital for a healthy nervous system and for the growth of red blood cells in bone marrow; food sources for vitamin B^{12} include yeast, milk, fish, eggs, and meat.

- **Vitamin C** allows the body's immune system to fight various medical conditions, strengthens body tissue, and improves the body's use of iron; food sources for vitamin C include a wide variety of fruits and vegetables.

- **Vitamin D** helps the body absorb calcium which strengthens bones and teeth; food sources for vitamin D include oily fish and dairy products.

- **Vitamin E** can help protect certain organs and tissues from various degenerative diseases; food sources for vitamin E include margarine, vegetables, eggs, and fish.

- **Vitamin K** is essential for bone formation and blood clotting; common food sources for vitamin K include leafy green vegetables.

- **Folic Acid** maintains healthy cells and blood; food sources for folic acid include nuts, fortified breads, leafy green vegetables, and whole grains.

It should be noted that it is possible to overdose on certain vitamins which become toxic if consumed in excess (e.g. vitamin A, D, E and K).

Like vitamins, minerals are chemicals that are required by the body to remain in good health. Because the human body does not manufacture these chemicals internally, we obtain them from food and other dietary sources. The more important minerals include:

- **Calcium** is needed for healthy bones, teeth, and muscles, but also helps the nervous system function; food sources for calcium include dry beans, peas, eggs, and dairy products.

- **Chromium** is helpful in regulating sugar levels in blood; food sources for chromium include egg yolks, raw sugar, cheese, nuts, beets, whole grains, and meat.

- **Fluoride** is used by the body to help prevent tooth decay and to reinforce bone strength; sources of fluoride include drinking water and certain brands of toothpaste.

- **Iodine** helps regulate the body's use of energy by synthesizing into the hormone thyroxine; food sources include leafy green vegetables, nuts, egg yolks, and red meat.

- **Iron** helps maintain muscles and the formation of red blood cells and certain proteins; food sources for iron include meat, dairy products, eggs, and leafy green vegetables.

- **Magnesium** is important for the production of DNA, as well as for healthy teeth, bones, muscles, and nerves; food sources for magnesium include dried fruit, dark green vegetables, nuts, and seafood.

- **Phosphorous** is used by the body to work with calcium to form bones and teeth; food sources for phosphorous include eggs, meat, cereals, and dairy products.

- **Selenium** primarily helps maintain normal heart and liver functions; food sources for selenium include wholegrain cereals, fish, meat, and dairy products.

- **Zinc** helps wounds heal, the formation of sperm, and encourage rapid growth and energy; food sources include dried beans, shellfish, eggs, and nuts.

The United States government periodically publishes recommended diets and consumption levels of the various elements of food. Again, the doctor may encourage deviations from the average official recommendation based on your child's specific condition. To learn more about basic dietary guidelines, visit the Web site: **http://www.health.gov/dietaryguidelines/**. Based on these guidelines, many foods are required to list the nutrition levels on the food's packaging. Labeling Requirements are listed at the following site maintained by the Food and Drug Administration: **http://www.cfsan.fda.gov/~dms/lab-cons.html**. When interpreting these requirements, the government recommends that consumers become familiar with the following abbreviations before reading FDA literature:[41]

- **DVs (Daily Values):** A new dietary reference term that will appear on the food label. It is made up of two sets of references, DRVs and RDIs.

- **DRVs (Daily Reference Values):** A set of dietary references that applies to fat, saturated fat, cholesterol, carbohydrate, protein, fiber, sodium, and potassium.

- **RDIs (Reference Daily Intakes):** A set of dietary references based on the Recommended Dietary Allowances for essential vitamins and minerals and, in selected groups, protein. The name "RDI" replaces the term "U.S. RDA."

- **RDAs (Recommended Dietary Allowances):** A set of estimated nutrient allowances established by the National Academy of Sciences. It is updated periodically to reflect current scientific knowledge.

---

[41] Adapted from the FDA: **http://www.fda.gov/fdac/special/foodlabel/dvs.html**.

What Are Dietary Supplements?[42]

Dietary supplements are widely available through many commercial sources, including health food stores, grocery stores, pharmacies, and by mail. Dietary supplements are provided in many forms including tablets, capsules, powders, gel-tabs, extracts, and liquids. Historically in the United States, the most prevalent type of dietary supplement was a multivitamin/mineral tablet or capsule that was available in pharmacies, either by prescription or "over the counter." Supplements containing strictly herbal preparations were less widely available. Currently in the United States, a wide array of supplement products are available, including vitamin, mineral, other nutrients, and botanical supplements as well as ingredients and extracts of animal and plant origin.

The Office of Dietary Supplements (ODS) of the National Institutes of Health is the official agency of the United States which has the expressed goal of acquiring "new knowledge to help prevent, detect, diagnose, and treat disease and disability, from the rarest genetic disorder to the common cold."[43] According to the ODS, dietary supplements can have an important impact on the prevention and management of medical conditions and on the maintenance of health.[44] The ODS notes that considerable research on the effects of dietary supplements has been conducted in Asia and Europe where the use of plant products, in particular, has a long tradition. However, the overwhelming majority of supplements have not been studied scientifically. To explore the role of dietary supplements in the improvement of health care, the ODS plans, organizes, and supports conferences, workshops, and symposia on scientific topics related to dietary supplements. The ODS often works in conjunction with other NIH Institutes and Centers, other government agencies, professional organizations, and public advocacy groups.

---

[42] This discussion has been adapted from the NIH: **http://ods.od.nih.gov/showpage.aspx?pageid=46**.

[43] Contact: The Office of Dietary Supplements, National Institutes of Health, Building 31, Room 1B29, 31 Center Drive, MSC 2086, Bethesda, Maryland 20892-2086, Tel: (301) 435-2920, Fax: (301) 480-1845, E-mail: ods@nih.gov.

[44] Adapted from **http://ods.od.nih.gov/showpage.aspx?pageid=2**. The Dietary Supplement Health and Education Act defines dietary supplements as "a product (other than tobacco) intended to supplement the diet that bears or contains one or more of the following dietary ingredients: a vitamin, mineral, amino acid, herb or other botanical; or a dietary substance for use to supplement the diet by increasing the total dietary intake; or a concentrate, metabolite, constituent, extract, or combination of any ingredient described above; and intended for ingestion in the form of a capsule, powder, softgel, or gelcap, and not represented as a conventional food or as a sole item of a meal or the diet."

To learn more about official information on dietary supplements, visit the ODS site at **http://dietary-supplements.info.nih.gov/**. Or contact:

The Office of Dietary Supplements
National Institutes of Health
Building 31, Room 1B29
31 Center Drive, MSC 2086
Bethesda, Maryland 20892-2086
Tel: (301) 435-2920
Fax: (301) 480-1845
E-mail: ods@nih.gov

Finding Studies on Infantile Spasms

The NIH maintains an office dedicated to nutrition and diet. The National Institutes of Health's Office of Dietary Supplements (ODS) offers a searchable bibliographic database called the IBIDS (International Bibliographic Information on Dietary Supplements). The IBIDS contains over 460,000 scientific citations and summaries about dietary supplements and nutrition as well as references to published international, scientific literature on dietary supplements such as vitamins, minerals, and botanicals.[45] IBIDS is available to the public free of charge through the ODS Internet page: **http://ods.od.nih.gov/databases/ibids.html**.

After entering the search area, you have three choices: (1) IBIDS Consumer Database, (2) Full IBIDS Database, or (3) Peer Reviewed Citations Only. We recommend that you start with the Consumer Database. While you may not find references for the topics that are of most interest to you, check back periodically as this database is frequently updated. More studies can be found by searching the Full IBIDS Database. Healthcare professionals and researchers generally use the third option, which lists peer-reviewed citations. In all cases, we suggest that you take advantage of the "Advanced Search" option that allows you to retrieve up to 100 fully explained references in a comprehensive format. Type "infantile spasms" (or synonyms) into the search box. To narrow the search, you can also select the "Title" field.

---

[45] Adapted from **http://ods.od.nih.gov**. IBIDS is produced by the Office of Dietary Supplements (ODS) at the National Institutes of Health to assist the public, healthcare providers, educators, and researchers in locating credible, scientific information on dietary supplements. IBIDS was developed and will be maintained through an interagency partnership with the Food and Nutrition Information Center of the National Agricultural Library, U.S. Department of Agriculture.

The following information is typical of that found when using the "Full IBIDS Database" when searching using "infantile spasms" (or a synonym):

- **A patient with infantile spasms and low homovanillic acid levels in cerebrospinal fluid: L-dopa dependent seizures?**
  Author(s): Department of Paediatrics, Tokyo Women's Medical College, Japan.
  Source: Sugie, H Sugie, Y Kato, N Fukuyama, Y Eur-J-Pediatr. 1989 June; 148(7): 667-8 0340-6199

- **A risk-benefit assessment of treatments for infantile spasms.**
  Author(s): Department of Neuropediatrics, Hjpital St Vincent de Paul, Paris, France. nabbout@genethon.fr
  Source: Nabbout, R Drug-Saf. 2001; 24(11): 813-28 0114-5916

- **ACTH activates rapid eye movement-related phasic inhibition during REM sleep in patients with infantile spasms.**
  Author(s): Department of Pediatrics, Faculty of Medicine, Tokyo Medical and Dental University, Japan.
  Source: Kohyama, J Shimohira, M Tanuma, N Hasegawa, T Iwakawa, Y Acta-Neurol-Scand. 2000 March; 101(3): 145-52 0001-6314

- **ACTH induced adrenal enlargement in infants treated for infantile spasms and acute cerebellar encephalopathy.**
  Author(s): Department of Radiology, Babies Hospital, New York, NY 10032.
  Source: Liebling, M S Starc, T J McAlister, W H Ruzal Shapiro, C B Abramson, S J Berdon, W E Pediatr-Radiol. 1993; 23(6): 454-6 0301-0449

- **ACTH treatment of infantile spasms: mechanisms of its effects in modulation of neuronal excitability.**
  Author(s): Departments of Pediatrics, Anatomy and Neurobiology, and Neurology, University of California, Irvine, Irvine, California 92697, USA.
  Source: Brunson, K L Avishai Eliner, S Baram, T Z Int-Rev-Neurobiol. 2002; 49: 185-97 0074-7742

- **Brainstem involvement in infantile spasms: a study employing brainstem evoked potentials and magnetic resonance imaging.**
  Author(s): Department of Pediatrics, School of Medicine, University of Tokushima, Japan.
  Source: Miyazaki, M Hashimoto, T Tayama, M Kuroda, Y Neuropediatrics. 1993 June; 24(3): 126-30 0174-304X

- **Cerebrospinal fluid corticotropin and cortisol are reduced in infantile spasms.**
  Author(s): Department of Neurology, University of Southern California, Los Angeles, USA.

Source: Baram, T Z Mitchell, W G Hanson, R A Snead, O C Horton, E J Pediatr-Neurol. 1995 September; 13(2): 108-10 0887-8994

- **Changes in CSF neurotransmitters in infantile spasms.**
  Author(s): Department of Psychology, San Diego State University, CA 92182.
  Source: Langlais, P J Wardlow, M L Yamamoto, H Pediatr-Neurol. 1991 Nov-December; 7(6): 440-5 0887-8994

- **Effects of ACTH on brain midline structures in infants with infantile spasms.**
  Author(s): Department of Pediatrics, Fukui Medical School, Japan.
  Source: Konishi, Y Hayakawa, K Kuriyama, M Saito, M Fujii, Y Sudo, M Pediatr-Neurol. 1995 September; 13(2): 134-6 0887-8994

- **Efficacy of the ketogenic diet for infantile spasms.**
  Author(s): Department of Neurology, Pediatric Epilepsy Center, Johns Hopkins Medical Institutions, Baltimore, Maryland, USA. ekossoff@jhmi.edu
  Source: Kossoff, Eric H Pyzik, Paula L McGrogan, Jane R Vining, Eileen P G Freeman, John M Pediatrics. 2002 May; 109(5): 780-3 1098-4275

- **Epidemiologic features of infantile spasms in Slovenia.**
  Author(s): Department of Child Neurology, University Children's Hospital, Ljubljana, Slovenia. zvonka.rener@mf.uni-lj.si
  Source: Primec, Zvonka Rener Kopac, Stefan Neubauer, David Epilepsia. 2002 February; 43(2): 183-7 0013-9580

- **Hyperkalemia as a late side effect of prolonged adrenocorticotropic hormone therapy for infantile spasms.**
  Author(s): Department of Pediatrics, Beilinson Medical Center, Petah Tiqva, Israel.
  Source: Zeharia, A Levy, Y Rachmel, A Nitzan, M Steinherz, R Helv-Paediatr-Acta. 1987 June; 42(5-6): 433-6 0018-022X

- **Infantile spasms and Lennox-Gastaut syndrome.**
  Author(s): Pediatric Epilepsy Center, St. Louis Children's Hospital, MO 63110-1093, USA. trevathan_e@kids.wustl.edu
  Source: Trevathan, E J-Child-Neurol. 2002 February; 17 Suppl 2: 2S9-2S22 0883-0738

- **Infantile spasms associated with proximal duplication of chromosome 15q.**
  Author(s): Division of Neurology, Children's Hospital of Philadelphia, Pennsylvania 19104, USA.
  Source: Bingham, P M Spinner, N B Sovinsky, L Zackai, E H Chance, P F Pediatr-Neurol. 1996 September; 15(2): 163-5 0887-8994

- **Infantile spasms with predominantly unilateral cerebral abnormalities.**
  Author(s): Department of Pediatrics, Tokushima University School of Medicine, Japan.
  Source: Miyazaki, M Hashimoto, T Omura, H Satomura, S Bando, N Yoshimoto, T Tayama, M Kuroda, Y Neuropediatrics. 1994 December; 25(6): 325-30 0174-304X

- **Infantile spasms.**
  Author(s): Pediatric Epilepsy Center, Washington University School of Medicine and St. Louis Children's Hospital, St. Louis, MO 63110-1093, USA.
  Source: Wong, M Trevathan, E Pediatr-Neurol. 2001 February; 24(2): 89-98 0887-8994

- **Infantile spasms--a clinical perspective.**
  Source: Low, P S J-Singapore-Paediatr-Soc. 1989; 31(3-4): 147-52 0037-5683

- **Lack of clinical-EEG effects of naloxone injection on infantile spasms.**
  Author(s): Department of Pediatrics, University of Modena, Italy.
  Source: Nalin, A Petraglia, F Genazzani, A R Frigieri, G Facchinetti, F Childs-Nerv-Syst. 1988 December; 4(6): 365-6 0256-7040

- **Long-term outcomes of conventional therapy for infantile spasms.**
  Author(s): Department of Neurology, Medical University of South Carolina, Charleston, USA.
  Source: Holden, K R Clarke, S L Griesemer, D A Seizure. 1997 June; 6(3): 201-5 1059-1311

- **Medical treatment of patients with infantile spasms.**
  Author(s): Adult and Pediatric Epilepsy Program and Department of Pediatrics American University of Beirut, Medical Center Beirut, Lebanon.
  Source: Mikati, Mohamad A Lepejian, Garine A Holmes, Gregory L Clin-Neuropharmacol. 2002 Mar-April; 25(2): 61-70 0362-5664

- **Neurosteroids and infantile spasms: the deoxycorticosterone hypothesis.**
  Author(s): Epilepsy Research Section, National Institute of Neurological Disorders and Stroke, National Institutes of Health, Bethesda, Maryland 20892, USA.
  Source: Rogawski, M A Reddy, D S Int-Rev-Neurobiol. 2002; 49: 199-219 0074-7742

- **Newer GABAergic agents for pharmacotherapy of infantile spasms.**
  Author(s): Department of Molecular Biomedical Sciences, North Carolina State University, College of Veterinary Medicine, Raleigh, NC 27606, USA. samba_reddy@ncsu.edu

Source: Reddy, D S Drugs-Today-(Barc). 2002 October; 38(10): 657-75 0025-7656

- **Oral high-dose phenobarbital therapy for early infantile epileptic encephalopathy.**
  Author(s): Department of Pediatrics, Tokyo Metropolitan Hachioji Children's Hospital, Hachioji, Tokyo, Japan.
  Source: Ozawa, Hiroshi Kawada, Yuko Noma, Seiji Sugai, Kenji Pediatr-Neurol. 2002 March; 26(3): 222-4 0887-8994

- **Randomized trial of vigabatrin in patients with infantile spasms.**
  Author(s): Dallas Pediatric Neurology Associates, The Center for Epilepsy Treatment, Medical City Dallas Hospital, Texas 75230, USA. RoyDElterman@aol.com
  Source: Elterman, R D Shields, W D Mansfield, K A Nakagawa, J Neurology. 2001 October 23; 57(8): 1416-21 0028-3878

- **Steroids or vigabatrin in the treatment of infantile spasms?**
  Author(s): Children's Hospital, University of Kuopio, Kuopio, Finland.
  Source: Riikonen, R S Pediatr-Neurol. 2000 November; 23(5): 403-8 0887-8994

- **Studies on CSF tryptophan metabolism in infantile spasms.**
  Author(s): Department of Pediatrics; St. Marianna University School of Medicine; Kawasaki, Japan.
  Source: Yamamoto, H Pediatr-Neurol. 1991 Nov-December; 7(6): 411-4 0887-8994

- **Therapeutic efficacy of ACTH in symptomatic infantile spasms with hypsarrhythmia.**
  Author(s): Division of Pediatric Neurology, University of Minnesota Medical School, Minneapolis, USA.
  Source: Sher, P K Sheikh, M R Pediatr-Neurol. 1993 Nov-December; 9(6): 451-6 0887-8994

- **Treatment of infantile spasms with valproic acid.**
  Source: Soetomenggolo, T S Paediatr-Indones. 1988 Jan-February; 28(1-2): 20-6 0030-9311

- **Vigabatrin for infantile spasms.**
  Author(s): Neurology Division, Childrens Hospital Los Angeles, Los Angeles, California 90027, USA.
  Source: Mitchell, W G Shah, N S Pediatr-Neurol. 2002 September; 27(3): 161-4 0887-8994

- **Vigabatrin in infantile spasms: preliminary result.**
  Author(s): Department of Pediatric Neurology, Faculty of Medicine, Ramathibodi Hospital, Mahidol University, Bangkok, Thailand.

Source: Visudtibhan, A Chiemchanya, S Visudhiphan, P Phusirimongkol, S J-Med-Assoc-Thai. 1999 October; 82(10): 1000-5 0125-2208

- **Vigabatrin in the treatment of infantile spasms.**
  Author(s): Department of Neurology, Children's Hospital of Michigan, Wayne State University, Detroit 48201, USA.
  Source: Koo, B Pediatr-Neurol. 1999 February; 20(2): 106-10 0887-8994

- **Vigabatrin therapy in infantile spasms.**
  Author(s): Department of Pediatrics, Faculty of Medicine Siriraj Hospital, Mahidol University, Bangkok, Thailand.
  Source: Kankirawatana, P Raksadawan, N Balangkura, K J-Med-Assoc-Thai. 2002 August; 85 Suppl 2: S778-83 0125-2208

- **Vitamin B6 and valproic acid in treatment of infantile spasms.**
  Author(s): Department of Pediatrics, Shimane Medical University, Izumo, Japan.
  Source: Ito, M Okuno, T Hattori, H Fujii, T Mikawa, H Pediatr-Neurol. 1991 Mar-April; 7(2): 91-6 0887-8994

Federal Resources on Nutrition

In addition to the IBIDS, the United States Department of Health and Human Services (HHS) and the United States Department of Agriculture (USDA) provide many sources of information on general nutrition and health. Recommended resources include:

- healthfinder®, HHS's gateway to health information, including diet and nutrition:
  http://www.healthfinder.gov/scripts/SearchContext.asp?topic=238&page=0

- The United States Department of Agriculture's Web site dedicated to nutrition information: **www.nutrition.gov**

- The Food and Drug Administration's Web site for federal food safety information: **www.foodsafety.gov**

- The National Action Plan on Overweight and Obesity sponsored by the United States Surgeon General:
  http://www.surgeongeneral.gov/topics/obesity/

- The Center for Food Safety and Applied Nutrition has an Internet site sponsored by the Food and Drug Administration and the Department of Health and Human Services: **http://vm.cfsan.fda.gov/**

- Center for Nutrition Policy and Promotion sponsored by the United States Department of Agriculture: **http://www.usda.gov/cnpp/**

- Food and Nutrition Information Center, National Agricultural Library sponsored by the United States Department of Agriculture: http://www.nal.usda.gov/fnic/
- Food and Nutrition Service sponsored by the United States Department of Agriculture: http://www.fns.usda.gov/fns/

Additional Web Resources

A number of additional Web sites offer encyclopedic information covering food and nutrition. The following is a representative sample:

- AOL: http://search.aol.com/cat.adp?id=174&layer=&from=subcats
- Family Village: http://www.familyvillage.wisc.edu/med_nutrition.html
- Google: http://directory.google.com/Top/Health/Nutrition/
- Open Directory Project: http://dmoz.org/Health/Nutrition/
- Yahoo.com: http://dir.yahoo.com/Health/Nutrition/
- WebMD®Health: http://my.webmd.com/nutrition
- WholeHealthMD.com: http://www.wholehealthmd.com/reflib/0,1529,,00.html

Vocabulary Builder

The following vocabulary builder defines words used in the references in this chapter that have not been defined in previous chapters:

Potassium: It is essential to the ability of muscle cells to contract. [NIH]

Wound: Any interruption, by violence or by surgery, in the continuity of the external surface of the body or of the surface of any internal organ. [NIH]

APPENDIX D. FINDING MEDICAL LIBRARIES

Overview

At a medical library you can find medical texts and reference books, consumer health publications, specialty newspapers and magazines, as well as medical journals. In this Appendix, we show you how to quickly find a medical library in your area.

Preparation

Before going to the library, highlight the references mentioned in this sourcebook that you find interesting. Focus on those items that are not available via the Internet, and ask the reference librarian for help with your search. He or she may know of additional resources that could be helpful to you. Most importantly, your local public library and medical libraries have Interlibrary Loan programs with the National Library of Medicine (NLM), one of the largest medical collections in the world. According to the NLM, most of the literature in the general and historical collections of the National Library of Medicine is available on interlibrary loan to any library. NLM's interlibrary loan services are only available to libraries. If you would like to access NLM medical literature, then visit a library in your area that can request the publications for you.[46]

---

[46] Adapted from the NLM: http://www.nlm.nih.gov/psd/cas/interlibrary.html.

Finding a Local Medical Library

The quickest method to locate medical libraries is to use the Internet-based directory published by the National Network of Libraries of Medicine (NN/LM). This network includes 4626 members and affiliates that provide many services to librarians, health professionals, and the public. To find a library in your area, simply visit **http://nnlm.gov/members/adv.html** or call 1-800-338-7657.

Medical Libraries in the U.S. and Canada

In addition to the NN/LM, the National Library of Medicine (NLM) lists a number of libraries with reference facilities that are open to the public. The following is the NLM's list and includes hyperlinks to each library's Web site. These Web pages can provide information on hours of operation and other restrictions. The list below is a small sample of libraries recommended by the National Library of Medicine (sorted alphabetically by name of the U.S. state or Canadian province where the library is located)[47]:

- **Alabama:** Health InfoNet of Jefferson County (Jefferson County Library Cooperative, Lister Hill Library of the Health Sciences), **http://www.uab.edu/infonet/**

- **Alabama:** Richard M. Scrushy Library (American Sports Medicine Institute)

- **Arizona:** Samaritan Regional Medical Center: The Learning Center (Samaritan Health System, Phoenix, Arizona), **http://www.samaritan.edu/library/bannerlibs.htm**

- **California:** Kris Kelly Health Information Center (St. Joseph Health System, Humboldt), **http://www.humboldt1.com/~kkhic/index.html**

- **California:** Community Health Library of Los Gatos, **http://www.healthlib.org/orgresources.html**

- **California:** Consumer Health Program and Services (CHIPS) (County of Los Angeles Public Library, Los Angeles County Harbor-UCLA Medical Center Library) - Carson, CA, **http://www.colapublib.org/services/chips.html**

- **California:** Gateway Health Library (Sutter Gould Medical Foundation)

- **California:** Health Library (Stanford University Medical Center), **http://www-med.stanford.edu/healthlibrary/**

---

[47] Abstracted from **http://www.nlm.nih.gov/medlineplus/libraries.html**.

- **California:** Patient Education Resource Center - Health Information and Resources (University of California, San Francisco), **http://sfghdean.ucsf.edu/barnett/PERC/default.asp**

- **California:** Redwood Health Library (Petaluma Health Care District), **http://www.phcd.org/rdwdlib.html**

- **California:** Los Gatos PlaneTree Health Library, **http://planetreesanjose.org/**

- **California:** Sutter Resource Library (Sutter Hospitals Foundation, Sacramento), **http://suttermedicalcenter.org/library/**

- **California:** Health Sciences Libraries (University of California, Davis), **http://www.lib.ucdavis.edu/healthsci/**

- **California:** ValleyCare Health Library & Ryan Comer Cancer Resource Center (ValleyCare Health System, Pleasanton), **http://gaelnet.stmarys-ca.edu/other.libs/gbal/east/vchl.html**

- **California:** Washington Community Health Resource Library (Fremont), **http://www.healthlibrary.org/**

- **Colorado:** William V. Gervasini Memorial Library (Exempla Healthcare), **http://www.saintjosephdenver.org/yourhealth/libraries/**

- **Connecticut:** Hartford Hospital Health Science Libraries (Hartford Hospital), **http://www.harthosp.org/library/**

- **Connecticut:** Healthnet: Connecticut Consumer Health Information Center (University of Connecticut Health Center, Lyman Maynard Stowe Library), **http://library.uchc.edu/departm/hnet/**

- **Connecticut:** Waterbury Hospital Health Center Library (Waterbury Hospital, Waterbury), **http://www.waterburyhospital.com/library/consumer.shtml**

- **Delaware:** Consumer Health Library (Christiana Care Health System, Eugene du Pont Preventive Medicine & Rehabilitation Institute, Wilmington), **http://www.christianacare.org/health_guide/health_guide_pmri_health_info.cfm**

- **Delaware:** Lewis B. Flinn Library (Delaware Academy of Medicine, Wilmington), **http://www.delamed.org/chls.html**

- **Georgia:** Family Resource Library (Medical College of Georgia, Augusta), **http://cmc.mcg.edu/kids_families/fam_resources/fam_res_lib/frl.htm**

- **Georgia:** Health Resource Center (Medical Center of Central Georgia, Macon), **http://www.mccg.org/hrc/hrchome.asp**

- **Hawaii:** Hawaii Medical Library: Consumer Health Information Service (Hawaii Medical Library, Honolulu), **http://hml.org/CHIS/**

- **Idaho:** DeArmond Consumer Health Library (Kootenai Medical Center, Coeur d'Alene), **http://www.nicon.org/DeArmond/index.htm**

- **Illinois:** Health Learning Center of Northwestern Memorial Hospital (Chicago), **http://www.nmh.org/health_info/hlc.html**

- **Illinois:** Medical Library (OSF Saint Francis Medical Center, Peoria), **http://www.osfsaintfrancis.org/general/library/**

- **Kentucky:** Medical Library - Services for Patients, Families, Students & the Public (Central Baptist Hospital, Lexington), **http://www.centralbap.com/education/community/library.cfm**

- **Kentucky:** University of Kentucky - Health Information Library (Chandler Medical Center, Lexington), **http://www.mc.uky.edu/PatientEd/**

- **Louisiana:** Alton Ochsner Medical Foundation Library (Alton Ochsner Medical Foundation, New Orleans), **http://www.ochsner.org/library/**

- **Louisiana:** Louisiana State University Health Sciences Center Medical Library-Shreveport, **http://lib-sh.lsuhsc.edu/**

- **Maine:** Franklin Memorial Hospital Medical Library (Franklin Memorial Hospital, Farmington), **http://www.fchn.org/fmh/lib.htm**

- **Maine:** Gerrish-True Health Sciences Library (Central Maine Medical Center, Lewiston), **http://www.cmmc.org/library/library.html**

- **Maine:** Hadley Parrot Health Science Library (Eastern Maine Healthcare, Bangor), **http://www.emh.org/hll/hpl/guide.htm**

- **Maine:** Maine Medical Center Library (Maine Medical Center, Portland), **http://www.mmc.org/library/**

- **Maine:** Parkview Hospital (Brunswick), **http://www.parkviewhospital.org/**

- **Maine:** Southern Maine Medical Center Health Sciences Library (Southern Maine Medical Center, Biddeford), **http://www.smmc.org/services/service.php3?choice=10**

- **Maine:** Stephens Memorial Hospital's Health Information Library (Western Maine Health, Norway), **http://www.wmhcc.org/Library/**

- **Manitoba, Canada:** Consumer & Patient Health Information Service (University of Manitoba Libraries), **http://www.umanitoba.ca/libraries/units/health/reference/chis.html**

- **Manitoba, Canada:** J.W. Crane Memorial Library (Deer Lodge Centre, Winnipeg), **http://www.deerlodge.mb.ca/crane_library/about.asp**

- **Maryland:** Health Information Center at the Wheaton Regional Library (Montgomery County, Dept. of Public Libraries, Wheaton Regional Library), **http://www.mont.lib.md.us/healthinfo/hic.asp**

- **Massachusetts:** Baystate Medical Center Library (Baystate Health System), **http://www.baystatehealth.com/1024/**

- **Massachusetts:** Boston University Medical Center Alumni Medical Library (Boston University Medical Center), **http://med-libwww.bu.edu/library/lib.html**

- **Massachusetts:** Lowell General Hospital Health Sciences Library (Lowell General Hospital, Lowell), **http://www.lowellgeneral.org/library/HomePageLinks/WWW.htm**

- **Massachusetts:** Paul E. Woodard Health Sciences Library (New England Baptist Hospital, Boston), **http://www.nebh.org/health_lib.asp**

- **Massachusetts:** St. Luke's Hospital Health Sciences Library (St. Luke's Hospital, Southcoast Health System, New Bedford), **http://www.southcoast.org/library/**

- **Massachusetts:** Treadwell Library Consumer Health Reference Center (Massachusetts General Hospital), **http://www.mgh.harvard.edu/library/chrcindex.html**

- **Massachusetts:** UMass HealthNet (University of Massachusetts Medical School, Worcester), **http://healthnet.umassmed.edu/**

- **Michigan:** Botsford General Hospital Library - Consumer Health (Botsford General Hospital, Library & Internet Services), **http://www.botsfordlibrary.org/consumer.htm**

- **Michigan:** Helen DeRoy Medical Library (Providence Hospital and Medical Centers), **http://www.providence-hospital.org/library/**

- **Michigan:** Marquette General Hospital - Consumer Health Library (Marquette General Hospital, Health Information Center), **http://www.mgh.org/center.html**

- **Michigan:** Patient Education Resouce Center - University of Michigan Cancer Center (University of Michigan Comprehensive Cancer Center, Ann Arbor), **http://www.cancer.med.umich.edu/learn/leares.htm**

- **Michigan:** Sladen Library & Center for Health Information Resources - Consumer Health Information (Detroit), **http://www.henryford.com/body.cfm?id=39330**

- **Montana:** Center for Health Information (St. Patrick Hospital and Health Sciences Center, Missoula)

- **National:** Consumer Health Library Directory (Medical Library Association, Consumer and Patient Health Information Section), http://caphis.mlanet.org/directory/index.html

- **National:** National Network of Libraries of Medicine (National Library of Medicine) - provides library services for health professionals in the United States who do not have access to a medical library, http://nnlm.gov/

- **National:** NN/LM List of Libraries Serving the Public (National Network of Libraries of Medicine), http://nnlm.gov/members/

- **Nevada:** Health Science Library, West Charleston Library (Las Vegas-Clark County Library District, Las Vegas), http://www.lvccld.org/special_collections/medical/index.htm

- **New Hampshire:** Dartmouth Biomedical Libraries (Dartmouth College Library, Hanover), http://www.dartmouth.edu/~biomed/resources.htmld/conshealth.htmld

- **New Jersey:** Consumer Health Library (Rahway Hospital, Rahway), http://www.rahwayhospital.com/library.htm

- **New Jersey:** Dr. Walter Phillips Health Sciences Library (Englewood Hospital and Medical Center, Englewood), http://www.englewoodhospital.com/links/index.htm

- **New Jersey:** Meland Foundation (Englewood Hospital and Medical Center, Englewood), http://www.geocities.com/ResearchTriangle/9360/

- **New York:** Choices in Health Information (New York Public Library) - NLM Consumer Pilot Project participant, http://www.nypl.org/branch/health/links.html

- **New York:** Health Information Center (Upstate Medical University, State University of New York, Syracuse), http://www.upstate.edu/library/hic/

- **New York:** Health Sciences Library (Long Island Jewish Medical Center, New Hyde Park), http://www.lij.edu/library/library.html

- **New York:** ViaHealth Medical Library (Rochester General Hospital), http://www.nyam.org/library/

- **Ohio:** Consumer Health Library (Akron General Medical Center, Medical & Consumer Health Library), http://www.akrongeneral.org/hwlibrary.htm

- **Oklahoma:** The Health Information Center at Saint Francis Hospital (Saint Francis Health System, Tulsa), **http://www.sfh-tulsa.com/services/healthinfo.asp**

- **Oregon:** Planetree Health Resource Center (Mid-Columbia Medical Center, The Dalles), **http://www.mcmc.net/phrc/**

- **Pennsylvania:** Community Health Information Library (Milton S. Hershey Medical Center, Hershey), **http://www.hmc.psu.edu/commhealth/**

- **Pennsylvania:** Community Health Resource Library (Geisinger Medical Center, Danville), **http://www.geisinger.edu/education/commlib.shtml**

- **Pennsylvania:** HealthInfo Library (Moses Taylor Hospital, Scranton), **http://www.mth.org/healthwellness.html**

- **Pennsylvania:** Hopwood Library (University of Pittsburgh, Health Sciences Library System, Pittsburgh), **http://www.hsls.pitt.edu/guides/chi/hopwood/index_html**

- **Pennsylvania:** Koop Community Health Information Center (College of Physicians of Philadelphia), **http://www.collphyphil.org/kooppg1.shtml**

- **Pennsylvania:** Learning Resources Center - Medical Library (Susquehanna Health System, Williamsport), **http://www.shscares.org/services/lrc/index.asp**

- **Pennsylvania:** Medical Library (UPMC Health System, Pittsburgh), **http://www.upmc.edu/passavant/library.htm**

- **Quebec, Canada:** Medical Library (Montreal General Hospital), **http://www.mghlib.mcgill.ca/**

- **South Dakota:** Rapid City Regional Hospital Medical Library (Rapid City Regional Hospital), **http://www.rcrh.org/Services/Library/Default.asp**

- **Texas:** Houston HealthWays (Houston Academy of Medicine-Texas Medical Center Library), **http://hhw.library.tmc.edu/**

- **Washington:** Community Health Library (Kittitas Valley Community Hospital), **http://www.kvch.com/**

- **Washington:** Southwest Washington Medical Center Library (Southwest Washington Medical Center, Vancouver), **http://www.swmedicalcenter.com/body.cfm?id=72**

APPENDIX E. SEIZURES AND EPILEPSY: HOPE THROUGH RESEARCH

Overview[48]

Few experiences match the drama of a convulsive seizure. A person having a severe seizure may cry out, fall to the floor unconscious, twitch or move uncontrollably, drool, or even lose bladder control. Within minutes, the attack is over, and the person regains consciousness but is exhausted and dazed. This is the image most people have when they hear the word epilepsy. However, this type of seizure—a generalized tonic-clonic seizure*—is only one kind of epilepsy. There are many other kinds, each with a different set of symptoms.

Epilepsy was one of the first brain disorders to be described. It was mentioned in ancient Babylon more than 3,000 years ago. The strange behavior caused by some seizures has contributed through the ages to many superstitions and prejudices. The word epilepsy is derived from the Greek word for "attack." People once thought that those with epilepsy were being visited by demons or gods. However, in 400 B.C., the early physician Hippocrates suggested that epilepsy was a disorder of the brain—and we now know that he was right.

Epilepsy is a brain disorder in which clusters of nerve cells, or neurons, in the brain sometimes signal abnormally. Neurons normally generate electrochemical impulses that act on other neurons, glands, and muscles to produce human thoughts, feelings, and actions. In epilepsy, the normal pattern of neuronal activity becomes disturbed, causing strange sensations,

---

[48] Adapted from The National Institute of Neurological Disorders and Stroke (NINDS): http://www.ninds.nih.gov/health_and_medical/pubs/seizures_and_epilepsy_htr.htm.

emotions, and behavior, or sometimes convulsions, muscle spasms, and loss of consciousness. During a seizure, neurons may fire as many as 500 times a second, much faster than the normal rate of about 80 times a second. In some people, this happens only occasionally; for others, it may happen up to hundreds of times a day.

More than 2 million people in the United States—about 1 in 100—have experienced an unprovoked seizure or been diagnosed with epilepsy. For about 80 percent of those diagnosed with epilepsy, seizures can be controlled with modern medicines and surgical techniques. However, about 20 percent of people with epilepsy will continue to experience seizures even with the best available treatment. Doctors call this situation intractable epilepsy. Having a seizure does not necessarily mean that a person has epilepsy. Only when a person has had two or more seizures is he or she considered to have epilepsy.

Epilepsy is not contagious and is not caused by mental illness or mental retardation. Some people with mental retardation may experience seizures, but seizures do not necessarily mean the person has or will develop mental impairment. Many people with epilepsy have normal or above-average intelligence. Famous people who are known or rumored to have had epilepsy include the Russian writer Dostoyevsky, the philosopher Socrates, the military general Napoleon, and the inventor of dynamite, Alfred Nobel, who established the Nobel prize. Several Olympic medalists and other athletes also have had epilepsy. Seizures sometimes do cause brain damage, particularly if they are severe. However, most seizures do not seem to have a detrimental effect on the brain. Any changes that do occur are usually subtle, and it is often unclear whether these changes are caused by the seizures themselves or by the underlying problem that caused the seizures.

While epilepsy cannot currently be cured, for some people it does eventually go away. One study found that children with idiopathic epilepsy, or epilepsy with an unknown cause, had a 68 to 92 percent chance of becoming seizure-free by 20 years after their diagnosis. The odds of becoming seizure-free are not as good for adults, or for children with severe epilepsy syndromes, but it is nonetheless possible that seizures may decrease or even stop over time. This is more likely if the epilepsy has been well-controlled by medication or if the person has had epilepsy surgery.

What Causes Epilepsy?

Epilepsy is a disorder with many possible causes. Anything that disturbs the normal pattern of neuron activity — from illness to brain damage to abnormal brain development — can lead to seizures.

Epilepsy may develop because of an abnormality in brain wiring, an imbalance of nerve signaling chemicals called neurotransmitters, or some combination of these factors. Researchers believe that some people with epilepsy have an abnormally high level of excitatory neurotransmitters that increase neuronal activity, while others have an abnormally low level of inhibitory neurotransmitters that decrease neuronal activity in the brain. Either situation can result in too much neuronal activity and cause epilepsy. One of the most-studied neurotransmitters that plays a role in epilepsy is GABA, or gamma-aminobutyric acid, which is an inhibitory neurotransmitter. Research on GABA has led to drugs that alter the amount of this neurotransmitter in the brain or change how the brain responds to it. Researchers also are studying excitatory neurotransmitters such as glutamate.

In some cases, the brain's attempts to repair itself after a head injury, stroke, or other problem may inadvertently generate abnormal nerve connections that lead to epilepsy. Abnormalities in brain wiring that occur during brain development also may disturb neuronal activity and lead to epilepsy.

Research has shown that the cell membrane that surrounds each neuron plays an important role in epilepsy. Cell membranes are crucial for neurons to generate electrical impulses. For this reason, researchers are studying details of the membrane structure, how molecules move in and out of membranes, and how the cell nourishes and repairs the membrane. A disruption in any of these processes may lead to epilepsy. Studies in animals have shown that, because the brain continually adapts to changes in stimuli, a small change in neuronal activity, if repeated, may eventually lead to full-blown epilepsy. Researchers are investigating whether this phenomenon, called kindling, may also occur in humans.

In some cases, epilepsy may result from changes in non-neuronal brain cells called glia. These cells regulate concentrations of chemicals in the brain that can affect neuronal signaling.

About half of all seizures have no known cause. However, in other cases, the seizures are clearly linked to infection, trauma, or other identifiable problems.

Genetic Factors

Research suggests that genetic abnormalities may be some of the most important factors contributing to epilepsy. Some types of epilepsy have been traced to an abnormality in a specific gene. Many other types of epilepsy tend to run in families, which suggests that genes influence epilepsy. Some researchers estimate that more than 500 genes could play a role in this disorder. However, it is increasingly clear that, for many forms of epilepsy, genetic abnormalities play only a partial role, perhaps by increasing a person's susceptibility to seizures that are triggered by an environmental factor.

Several types of epilepsy have now been linked to defective genes for ion channels, the "gates" that control the flow of ions in and out of cells and regulate neuron signaling. Another gene, which is missing in people with progressive myoclonus epilepsy, codes for a protein called cystatin B. This protein regulates enzymes that break down other proteins. Another gene, which is altered in a severe form of epilepsy called LaFora disease, has been linked to a gene that helps to break down carbohydrates.

While abnormal genes sometimes cause epilepsy, they also may influence the disorder in subtler ways. For example, one study showed that many people with epilepsy have an abnormally active version of a gene that increases resistance to drugs. This may help explain why anticonvulsant drugs do not work for some people. Genes also may control other aspects of the body's response to medications and each person's susceptibility to seizures, or seizure threshold. Abnormalities in the genes that control neuronal migration—a critical step in brain development— can lead to areas of misplaced or abnormally formed neurons, or dysplasia, in the brain that can cause epilepsy. In some cases, genes may contribute to development of epilepsy even in people with no family history of the disorder. These people may have a newly developed abnormality, or mutation, in an epilepsy-related gene.

Other Disorders

In many cases, epilepsy develops as a result of brain damage from other disorders. For example, brain tumors, alcoholism, and Alzheimer's disease frequently lead to epilepsy because they alter the normal workings of the brain. Strokes, heart attacks, and other conditions that deprive the brain of oxygen also can cause epilepsy in some cases. About 32 percent of all newly developed epilepsy in elderly people appears to be due to cerebrovascular disease, which reduces the supply of oxygen to brain cells. Meningitis, AIDS, viral encephalitis, and other infectious diseases can lead to epilepsy, as can hydrocephalus—a condition in which excess fluid builds up in the brain. Epilepsy also can result from intolerance to wheat gluten (known as celiac disease), or from a parasitic infection of the brain called neurocysticercosis. Seizures may stop once these disorders are treated successfully. However, the odds of becoming seizure-free after the primary disorder is treated are uncertain and vary depending on the type of disorder, the brain region that is affected, and how much brain damage occurred prior to treatment.

Epilepsy is associated with a variety of developmental and metabolic disorders, including cerebral palsy, neurofibromatosis, pyruvate deficiency, tuberous sclerosis, Landau-Kleffner syndrome, and autism. Epilepsy is just one of a set of symptoms commonly found in people with these disorders.

Head Injury

In some cases, head injury can lead to seizures or epilepsy. Safety measures such as wearing seat belts in cars and using helmets when riding a motorcycle or playing competitive sports can protect people from epilepsy and other problems that result from head injury.

Prenatal Injury and Developmental Problems

The developing brain is susceptible to many kinds of injury. Maternal infections, poor nutrition, and oxygen deficiencies are just some of the conditions that may take a toll on the brain of a developing baby. These conditions may lead to cerebral palsy, which often is associated with epilepsy, or they may cause epilepsy that is unrelated to any other disorders. About 20 percent of seizures in children are due to cerebral palsy or other neurological abnormalities. Abnormalities in genes that control development also may contribute to epilepsy. Advanced brain imaging has revealed that some cases of epilepsy that occur with no obvious cause may be associated with areas of dysplasia in the brain that probably develop before birth.

Poisoning

Seizures can result from exposure to lead, carbon monoxide, and many other poisons. They also can result from exposure to street drugs and from overdoses of antidepressants and other medications.

Seizure Triggers

Seizures are often triggered by factors such as lack of sleep, alcohol consumption, stress, or hormonal changes associated with the menstrual cycle. These seizure triggers do not cause epilepsy but can provoke first seizures or cause breakthrough seizures in people who otherwise experience good seizure control with their medication. Sleep deprivation in particular is a universal and powerful trigger of seizures. For this reason, people with epilepsy should make sure to get enough sleep and should try to stay on a regular sleep schedule as much as possible. For some people, light flashing at a certain speed or the flicker of a computer monitor can trigger a seizure; this problem is called photosensitive epilepsy. Smoking cigarettes also can trigger seizures. The nicotine in cigarettes acts on receptors for the excitatory neurotransmitter acetylcholine in the brain, which increases neuronal firing. Seizures are not triggered by sexual activity except in very rare instances.

What Are the Different Kinds of Seizures?

Doctors have described more than 30 different types of seizures. Seizures are divided into two major categories — partial seizures and generalized seizures. However, there are many different types of seizures in each of these categories.

Partial Seizures

Partial seizures occur in just one part of the brain. About 60 percent of people with epilepsy have partial seizures. These seizures are frequently described by the area of the brain in which they originate. For example, someone might be diagnosed with partial frontal lobe seizures.

In a simple partial seizure, the person will remain conscious but may experience unusual feelings or sensations that can take many forms. The person may experience sudden and unexplainable feelings of joy, anger, sadness, or nausea. He or she also may hear, smell, taste, see, or feel things that are not real.

In a complex partial seizure, the person has a change in or loss of consciousness. His or her consciousness may be altered, producing a dreamlike experience. People having a complex partial seizure may display strange, repetitious behaviors such as blinks, twitches, mouth movements, or even walking in a circle. These repetitious movements are called automatisms. They also may fling objects across the room or strike out at walls or furniture as though they are angry or afraid. These seizures usually last just a few seconds.

Some people with partial seizures, especially complex partial seizures, may experience auras—unusual sensations that warn of an impending seizure. These auras are actually simple partial seizures in which the person maintains consciousness. The symptoms an individual person has, and the progression of those symptoms, tends to be stereotyped, or similar every time.

The symptoms of partial seizures can easily be confused with other disorders. For instance, the dreamlike perceptions associated with a complex partial seizure may be misdiagnosed as migraine headaches, which also can cause a dreamlike state. The strange behavior and sensations caused by partial seizures also can be mistaken for symptoms of narcolepsy, fainting, or even mental illness. It may take many tests and careful monitoring by a knowledgeable physician to tell the difference between epilepsy and other disorders.

Generalized Seizures

Generalized seizures are a result of abnormal neuronal activity in many parts of the brain. These seizures may cause loss of consciousness, falls, or massive muscle spasms.

There are many kinds of generalized seizures. In absence seizures, the person may appear to be staring into space and/or have jerking or twitching muscles. These seizures are sometimes referred to as petit mal seizures, which is an older term. Tonic seizures cause stiffening of muscles of the body, generally those in the back, legs, and arms. Clonic seizures cause repeated jerking movements of muscles on both sides of the body. Myoclonic seizures cause jerks or twitches of the upper body, arms, or legs. Atonic seizures cause a loss of normal muscle tone. The affected person will fall down or may nod his or her head involuntarily. Tonic-clonic seizures cause a mixture of symptoms, including stiffening of the body and repeated jerks of the arms and/or legs as well as loss of consciousness. Tonic-clonic seizures are sometimes referred to by an older term: grand mal seizures.

Not all seizures can be easily defined as either partial or generalized. Some people have seizures that begin as partial seizures but then spread to the entire brain. Other people may have both types of seizures but with no clear pattern.

Society's lack of understanding about the many different types of seizures is one of the biggest problems for people with epilepsy. People who witness a non-convulsive seizure often find it difficult to understand that behavior which looks deliberate is not under the person's control. In some cases, this has led to the affected person being arrested, sued, or placed in a mental institution. To combat these problems, people everywhere need to understand the many different types of seizures and how they may appear.

What Are the Different Kinds of Epilepsy?

Just as there are many different kinds of seizures, there are many different kinds of epilepsy. Doctors have identified hundreds of different epilepsy syndromes—disorders characterized by a specific set of symptoms that include epilepsy. Some of these syndromes appear to be hereditary. For other syndromes, the cause is unknown. Epilepsy syndromes are frequently described by their symptoms or by where in the brain they originate. People should discuss the implications of their type of epilepsy with their doctors to understand the full range of symptoms, the possible treatments, and the prognosis.

People with absence epilepsy have repeated absence seizures that cause momentary lapses of consciousness. These seizures almost always begin in childhood or adolescence, and they tend to run in families, suggesting that they may be at least partially due to a defective gene or genes. Some people with absence seizures have purposeless movements during their seizures, such as a jerking arm or rapidly blinking eyes. Others have no noticeable symptoms except for brief times when they are "out of it." Immediately after a seizure, the person can resume whatever he or she was doing. However, these seizures may occur so frequently that the person cannot concentrate in school or other situations. Childhood absence epilepsy usually stops when the child reaches puberty. Absence seizures usually have no lasting effect on intelligence or other brain functions.

Psychomotor Epilepsy

Psychomotor epilepsy is another term for recurrent partial seizures, especially seizures of the temporal lobe. The term psychomotor refers to the strange sensations, emotions, and behavior seen with these seizures.

Temporal Lobe Epilepsy

Temporal lobe epilepsy, or TLE, is the most common epilepsy syndrome with partial seizures. These seizures are often associated with auras. TLE often begins in childhood. Research has shown that repeated temporal lobe seizures can cause a brain structure called the hippocampus to shrink over time. The hippocampus is important for memory and learning. While it may take years of temporal lobe seizures for measurable hippocampal damage to occur, this finding underlines the need to treat TLE early and as effectively as possible.

Frontal Lobe Epilepsy

Frontal lobe epilepsy usually involves a cluster of short seizures with a sudden onset and termination. There are many subtypes of frontal lobe seizures. The symptoms depend on where in the frontal lobe the seizures occur.

Occipital Lobe Epilepsy

Occipital lobe epilepsy usually begins with visual hallucinations, rapid eye blinking, or other eye-related symptoms. Otherwise, it resembles temporal or frontal lobe epilepsy.

The symptoms of parietal lobe epilepsy closely resemble those of other types of epilepsy. This may reflect the fact that parietal lobe seizures tend to spread to other areas of the brain.

Other Types of Epilepsy

There are many other types of epilepsy, each with its own characteristic set of symptoms. Many of these, including Lennox-Gastaut syndrome and Rasmussen's encephalitis, begin in childhood. Children with Lennox-Gastaut syndrome have severe epilepsy with several different types of seizures, including atonic seizures, which cause sudden falls and are also called drop attacks. This severe form of epilepsy can be very difficult to treat effectively. Rasmussen's encephalitis is a progressive type of epilepsy in which half of the brain shows continual inflammation. It sometimes is treated with a radical surgical procedure called hemispherectomy (see the section on Surgery). Some childhood epilepsy syndromes, such as childhood absence epilepsy, tend to go into remission or stop entirely during adolescence, whereas other syndromes such as juvenile myoclonic epilepsy are usually present for life once they develop. Seizure syndromes do not always appear in childhood. For example, Ramsay Hunt syndrome type II is a rare and severe progressive type of epilepsy that generally begins in early adulthood and leads to reduced muscle coordination and cognitive abilities in addition to seizures.

Benign Epilepsy Syndromes

Epilepsy syndromes that do not seem to impair cognitive functions or development are often described as benign. Benign epilepsy syndromes include benign infantile encephalopathy and benign neonatal convulsions. Other syndromes, such as early myoclonic encephalopathy, include neurological and developmental problems. However, these problems may be caused by underlying neurodegenerative processes rather than by the seizures. Epilepsy syndromes in which the seizures and/or the person's cognitive or motor abilities get worse over time are called progressive epilepsy.

Infantile Epilepsy

Several types of epilepsy begin in infancy. The most common type of infantile epilepsy is infantile spasms, clusters of seizures that usually begin before the age of 6 months. During these seizures the infant may bend and cry out. Anticonvulsant drugs often do not work for infantile spasms, but the seizures can be treated with ACTH (adrenocorticotropic hormone) or prednisone.

When Are Seizures Not Epilepsy?

While any seizure is cause for concern, having a seizure does not by itself mean a person has epilepsy. First seizures, febrile seizures, nonepileptic events, and eclampsia are examples of seizures that may not be associated with epilepsy.

First Seizures

Many people have a single seizure at some point in their lives. Often these seizures occur in reaction to anesthesia or a strong drug, but they also may be unprovoked, meaning that they occur without any obvious triggering factor. Unless the person has suffered brain damage or there is a family history of epilepsy or other neurological abnormalities, these single seizures usually are not followed by additional seizures. One recent study that followed patients for an average of 8 years found that only 33 percent of people have a second seizure within 4 years after an initial seizure. People who did not have a second seizure within that time remained seizure-free for the rest of the study. For people who did have a second seizure, the risk of a third seizure was about 73 percent on average by the end of 4 years.

When someone has experienced a first seizure, the doctor will usually order an electroencephalogram, or EEG, to determine what type of seizure the person may have had and if there are any detectable abnormalities in the person's brain waves. The doctor also may order brain scans to identify abnormalities that may be visible in the brain. These tests may help the doctor decide whether or not to treat the person with antiepileptic drugs. In some cases, drug treatment after the first seizure may help prevent future seizures and epilepsy. However, the drugs also can cause detrimental side effects, so doctors prescribe them only when they feel the benefits outweigh the risks. Evidence suggests that it may be beneficial to begin anticonvulsant medication once a person has had a second seizure, as the chance of future seizures increases significantly after this occurs.

Febrile Seizures

Sometimes a child will have a seizure during the course of an illness with a high fever. These seizures are called febrile seizures (febrile is derived from the Latin word for "fever") and can be very alarming to the parents and other caregivers. In the past, doctors usually prescribed a course of anticonvulsant drugs following a febrile seizure in the hope of preventing epilepsy. However, most children who have a febrile seizure do not develop epilepsy, and long-term use of anticonvulsant drugs in children may damage the developing brain or cause other detrimental side effects. Experts at a 1980 consensus conference coordinated by the National Institutes of Health concluded that preventive treatment after a febrile seizure is generally not warranted unless certain other conditions are present: a family history of epilepsy, signs of nervous system impairment prior to the seizure, or a relatively prolonged or complicated seizure. The risk of subsequent non-febrile seizures is only 2 to 3 percent unless one of these factors is present.

Researchers have now identified several different genes that influence the risk of febrile seizures in certain families. Studying these genes may lead to new understanding of how febrile seizures occur and perhaps point to ways of preventing them.

Nonepileptic Events

Sometimes people appear to have seizures, even though their brains show no seizure activity. This type of phenomenon has various names, including nonepileptic events and pseudoseizures. Both of these terms essentially mean something that looks like a seizure but isn't one. Nonepileptic events that are psychological in origin may be referred to as psychogenic seizures. Psychogenic seizures may indicate dependence, a need for attention, avoidance of stressful situations, or specific psychiatric conditions. Some people with epilepsy have psychogenic seizures in addition to their epileptic seizures. Other people who have psychogenic seizures do not have epilepsy at all. Psychogenic seizures cannot be treated in the same way as epileptic seizures. Instead, they are often treated by mental health specialists.

Other nonepileptic events may be caused by narcolepsy, Tourette syndrome, cardiac arrhythmia, and other medical conditions with symptoms that resemble seizures. Because symptoms of these disorders can look very much like epileptic seizures, they are often mistaken for epilepsy. Distinguishing between true epileptic seizures and nonepileptic events can be very difficult and requires a thorough medical assessment, careful monitoring, and knowledgeable health professionals. Improvements in brain scanning and monitoring technology may improve diagnosis of nonepileptic events in the future.

Eclampsia

Eclampsia is a life-threatening condition that can develop in pregnant women. Its symptoms include sudden elevations of blood pressure and seizures. Pregnant women who develop unexpected seizures should be rushed to a hospital immediately. Eclampsia can be treated in a hospital setting and usually does not result in additional seizures or epilepsy once the pregnancy is over.

How Is Epilepsy Diagnosed?

Doctors have developed a number of different tests to determine whether a person has epilepsy and, if so, what kind of seizures the person has. In some cases, people may have symptoms that look very much like a seizure but in fact are nonepileptic events caused by other disorders. Even doctors may not be able to tell the difference between these disorders and epilepsy without close observation and intensive testing.

EEG Monitoring

An EEG records brain waves detected by electrodes placed on the scalp. This is the most common diagnostic test for epilepsy and can detect abnormalities in the brain's electrical activity. People with epilepsy frequently have changes in their normal pattern of brain waves, even when they are not experiencing a seizure. While this type of test can be very useful in diagnosing epilepsy, it is not foolproof. Some people continue to show normal brain wave patterns even after they have experienced a seizure. In other cases, the unusual brain waves are generated deep in the brain where the EEG is unable to detect them. Many people who do not have epilepsy also show some unusual brain activity on an EEG. Whenever possible, an EEG should be performed within 24 hours of a patient's first seizure. Ideally, EEGs should be performed while the patient is sleeping as well as when he or she is awake, because brain activity during sleep is often quite different than at other times.

Video monitoring is often used in conjunction with EEG to determine the nature of a person's seizures. It also can be used in some cases to rule out other disorders such as cardiac arrhythmia or narcolepsy that may look like epilepsy.

In some cases, doctors may use an experimental diagnostic technique called a magnetoencephalogram, or MEG. MEG detects the magnetic signals generated by neurons to allow doctors to monitor brain activity at different points in the brain over time, revealing different brain functions. While MEG is similar in concept to EEG, it does not require electrodes and it can detect signals from deeper in the brain than an EEG.

Brain Scans

One of the most important ways of diagnosing epilepsy is through the use of brain scans. The most commonly used brain scans include CT (computed tomography), PET (positron emission tomography) and MRI (magnetic resonance imaging). CT and MRI scans reveal the structure of the brain, which can be useful for identifying brain tumors, cysts, and other structural abnormalities. PET and an adapted kind of MRI called functional MRI (fMRI) can be used to monitor the brain's activity and detect abnormalities in how it works. SPECT (single photon emission computed tomography) is a relatively new kind of brain scan that is sometimes used to locate seizure foci in the brain. Doctors also are experimenting with brain scans called magnetic resonance spectroscopy (MRS) that can detect abnormalities in the brain's biochemical processes, and with near-infrared spectroscopy, a technique that can detect oxygen levels in brain tissue.

Medical History

Taking a detailed medical history, including symptoms and duration of the seizures, is still one of the best methods available to determine if a person has epilepsy and what kind of seizures they have. The doctor will ask questions about the seizures and any past illnesses or other symptoms a person may have had. Since people who have suffered a seizure often do not remember what happened, caregivers' accounts of the seizure are vital to this evaluation.

Blood Tests

Doctors often take blood samples for testing, particularly when they are examining a child. These blood samples are often screened for metabolic or genetic disorders that may be associated with the seizures. They also may be used to check for underlying problems such as infections, lead poisoning, anemia, and diabetes that may be causing or triggering the seizures.

Developmental, Neurological, and Behavioral Tests

Doctors often use tests devised to measure motor abilities, behavior, and intellectual capacity as a way to determine how the epilepsy is affecting that person. These tests also can provide clues about what kind of epilepsy the person has.

Can Epilepsy Be Prevented?

Many cases of epilepsy can be prevented by wearing seatbelts and bicycle helmets, putting children in car seats, and other measures that prevent head injury and other trauma. Prescribing medication after first or second seizures or febrile seizures also may help prevent epilepsy in some cases. Good prenatal care, including treatment of high blood pressure and infections during pregnancy, can prevent brain damage in the developing baby that may lead to epilepsy and other neurological problems later. Treating cardiovascular disease, high blood pressure, infections, and other disorders that can affect the brain during adulthood and aging also may prevent many cases of epilepsy. Finally, identifying the genes for many neurological disorders can provide opportunities for genetic screening and prenatal diagnosis that may ultimately prevent many cases of epilepsy.

How Can Epilepsy Be Treated?

Accurate diagnosis of the type of epilepsy a person has is crucial for finding an effective treatment. There are many different ways to treat epilepsy. Currently available treatments can control seizures at least some of the time in about 80 percent of people with epilepsy. However, another 20 percent — about 600,000 people with epilepsy in the United States — have intractable seizures, and another 400,000 feel they get inadequate relief from available treatments. These statistics make it clear that improved treatments are desperately needed.

Doctors who treat epilepsy come from many different fields of medicine. They include neurologists, pediatricians, pediatric neurologists, internists, and family physicians, as well as neurosurgeons and doctors called epileptologists who specialize in treating epilepsy. People who need specialized or intensive care for epilepsy may be treated at large medical centers and neurology clinics at hospitals, or by neurologists in private practice. Many epilepsy treatment centers are associated with university hospitals that perform research in addition to providing medical care.

Once epilepsy is diagnosed, it is important to begin treatment as soon as possible. Research suggests that medication and other treatments may be less successful in treating epilepsy once seizures and their consequences become established.

Medications

By far the most common approach to treating epilepsy is to prescribe antiepileptic drugs. The first effective antiepileptic drugs were bromides, introduced by an English physician named Sir Charles Locock in 1857. He noticed that bromides had a sedative effect and seemed to reduce seizures in some patients. More than 20 different antiepileptic drugs are now on the market, all with different benefits and side effects. The choice of which drug to prescribe, and at what dosage, depends on many different factors, including the type of seizures a person has, the person's lifestyle and age, how frequently the seizures occur, and, for a woman, the likelihood that she will become pregnant. People with epilepsy should follow their doctor's advice and share any concerns they may have regarding their medication.

Doctors seeing a patient with newly developed epilepsy often prescribe carbamazapine, valproate, or phenytoin first, unless the epilepsy is a type that is known to require a different kind of treatment. For absence seizures, ethosuximide is often the primary treatment. Other commonly prescribed drugs include clonazepam, phenobarbital, and primidone. In recent years, a number of new drugs have become available. These include tiagabine, lamotrigine, gabapentin, topiramate, levetiracetam, felbamate, and zonisamide, as well as oxcarbazepine, a drug that is similar to carbamazapine but has fewer side effects. These new drugs may have advantages for many patients. Other drugs are used in combination with one of the standard drugs or for intractable seizures that do not respond to other medications. A few drugs, such as fosphenytoin, are approved for use only in hospital settings to treat specific problems such as status epilepticus (see section, "Are There Special Risks Associated With Epilepsy?"). For people with stereotyped recurrent severe seizures that can be easily recognized by the person's family, the drug diazepam is now available as a gel that can be administered rectally by a family member. This method of drug delivery may be able to stop prolonged seizures before they develop into status epilepticus.

For most people with epilepsy, seizures can be controlled with just one drug at the optimal dosage. Combining medications usually amplifies side effects such as fatigue and decreased appetite, so doctors usually prescribe monotherapy, or the use of just one drug, whenever possible. Combinations of drugs are sometimes prescribed if monotherapy fails to effectively control a patient's seizures.

The number of times a person needs to take medication each day is usually determined by the drug's half-life, or the time it takes for half the drug dose to be metabolized or broken down into other substances in the body. Some drugs, such as phenytoin and phenobarbital, only need to be taken once a day, while others such as valproate must be taken more frequently.

Most side effects of antiepileptic drugs are relatively minor, such as fatigue, dizziness, or weight gain. However, severe and life-threatening side effects such as allergic reactions can occur. Epilepsy medication also may predispose people to developing depression or psychoses. People with epilepsy should consult a doctor immediately if they develop any kind of rash while on medication, or if they find themselves depressed or otherwise unable to think in a rational manner. Other danger signs that should be discussed with a doctor immediately are extreme fatigue, staggering or other movement problems, and slurring of words. People with epilepsy should be aware that their epilepsy medication can interact with many other drugs in potentially harmful ways. For this reason, people with epilepsy should always tell doctors who treat them which medications they are taking. Women also should know that some antiepileptic drugs can interfere with the effectiveness of oral contraceptives, and they should discuss this possibility with their doctors.

Since people can become more sensitive to medications as they age, they should have their blood levels of medication checked occasionally to see if the dose needs to be adjusted. The effects of a particular medication also sometimes wear off over time, leading to an increase in seizures if the dose is not adjusted. People should know that some citrus fruit, in particular grapefruit juice, may interfere with breakdown of many drugs. This can cause too much of the drug to build up in their bodies, often worsening the side effects.

Tailoring the Dosage of Antiepileptic Drugs

When a person starts a new epilepsy drug, it is important to tailor the dosage to achieve the best results. People's bodies react to medications in very different and sometimes unpredictable ways, so it may take some time to find the right drug at the right dose to provide optimal control of seizures while minimizing side effects. A drug that has no effect or very bad side effects at one dose may work very well at another dose. Doctors will usually prescribe a low dose of the new drug initially and monitor blood levels of the drug to determine when the best possible dose has been reached.

Generic versions are available for many antiepileptic drugs. The chemicals in generic drugs are exactly the same as in the brand-name drugs, but they may be absorbed or processed differently in the body because of the way they are prepared. Therefore, patients should always check with their doctors before switching to a generic version of their medication.

Discontinuing Medication

Some doctors will advise people with epilepsy to discontinue their antiepileptic drugs after two years have passed without a seizure. Others feel it is better to wait for four to five years. Discontinuing medication should only be done with a doctor's advice and supervision. It is very important to continue taking epilepsy medication for as long as the doctor prescribes it. People also should ask the doctor or pharmacist ahead of time what they should do if they miss a dose. Discontinuing medication without a doctor's advice is one of the major reasons people who have been seizure-free begin having new seizures. Seizures that result from suddenly stopping medication can be very serious and can lead to status epilepticus. Furthermore, there is some evidence that uncontrolled seizures trigger changes in neurons that can make it more difficult to treat the seizures in the future.

The chance that a person will eventually be able to discontinue medication varies depending on the person's age and his or her type of epilepsy. More than half of children who go into remission with medication can eventually stop their medication without having new seizures. One study showed that 68 percent of adults who had been seizure-free for 2 years before stopping medication were able to do so without having more seizures and 75 percent could successfully discontinue medication if they had been seizure-free for 3 years. However, the odds of successfully stopping medication are not as good for people with a family history of epilepsy, those who need multiple medications, those with partial seizures, and those who continue to have abnormal EEG results while on medication.

Surgery

When seizures cannot be adequately controlled by medications, doctors may recommend that the person be evaluated for surgery. Most surgery for epilepsy is performed by teams of doctors at medical centers. To decide if a person may benefit from surgery, doctors consider the type or types of seizures he or she has. They also take into account the brain region involved and how important that region is for everyday behavior. Surgeons usually avoid operating in areas of the brain that are necessary for speech, language, hearing, or other important abilities. Doctors may perform tests such as a Wada test (administration of the drug amobarbitol into the carotid artery) to find areas of the brain that control speech and memory. They often monitor the patient intensively prior to surgery in order to pinpoint the exact location in the brain where seizures begin. They also may use implanted electrodes to record brain activity from the surface of the brain. This yields better information than an external EEG.

A 1990 National Institutes of Health consensus conference on surgery for epilepsy concluded that there are three broad categories of epilepsy that can be treated successfully with surgery. These include partial seizures, seizures that begin as partial seizures before spreading to the rest of the brain, and unilateral multifocal epilepsy with infantile hemiplegia (such as Rasmussen's encephalitis). Doctors generally recommend surgery only after patients have tried two or three different medications without success, or if there is an identifiable brain lesion — a damaged or abnormally functioning area — believed to cause the seizures.

If a person is considered a good candidate for surgery and has seizures that cannot be controlled with available medication, experts generally agree that surgery should be performed as early as possible. It can be difficult for a person who has had years of seizures to fully re-adapt to a seizure-free life if the surgery is successful. The person may never have had an opportunity to develop independence and he or she may have had difficulties with school and work that could have been avoided with earlier treatment. Surgery should always be performed with support from rehabilitation specialists and counselors who can help the person deal with the many psychological, social, and employment issues he or she may face.

While surgery can significantly reduce or even halt seizures for some people, it is important to remember that any kind of surgery carries some amount of risk (usually small). Surgery for epilepsy does not always successfully reduce seizures and it can result in cognitive or personality changes, even in people who are excellent candidates for surgery. Patients should ask their surgeon about his or her experience, success rates, and complication rates with the procedure they are considering.

Even when surgery completely ends a person's seizures, it is important to continue taking seizure medication for some time to give the brain time to re-adapt. Doctors generally recommend medication for 2 years after a successful operation to avoid new seizures.

Surgery to Treat Underlying Conditions

In cases where seizures are caused by a brain tumor, hydrocephalus, or other conditions that can be treated with surgery, doctors may operate to treat these underlying conditions. In many cases, once the underlying condition is successfully treated, a person's seizures will stop as well.

Surgery to Remove a Seizure Focus

The most common type of surgery for epilepsy is removal of a seizure focus, or small area of the brain where seizures originate. This type of surgery, which doctors may refer to as a lobectomy or lesionectomy, is appropriate only for partial seizures that originate in just one area of the brain. In general, people have a better chance of becoming seizure-free after surgery if they have a small, well-defined seizure focus. Lobectomies have a 55-70 percent success rate when the type of epilepsy and the seizure focus is well-defined. The most common type of lobectomy is a temporal lobe resection, which is performed for people with temporal lobe epilepsy. Temporal lobe resection leads to a significant reduction or complete cessation of seizures about 70 - 90 percent of the time.

Multiple Subpial Transection

When seizures originate in part of the brain that cannot be removed, surgeons may perform a procedure called a multiple subpial transection. In this type of operation, which was first described in 1989, surgeons make a series of cuts that are designed to prevent seizures from spreading into other parts of the brain while leaving the person's normal abilities intact. About 70 percent of patients who undergo a multiple subpial transection have satisfactory improvement in seizure control.

Corpus Callosotomy

Corpus callosotomy, Corpus callosotomy, or severing the network of neural connections between the right and left halves, or hemispheres, of the brain, is done primarily in children with severe seizures that start in one half of the brain and spread to the other side. Corpus callosotomy can end drop attacks and other generalized seizures. However, the procedure does not stop seizures in the side of the brain where they originate, and these partial seizures may even increase after surgery.

Hemispherectomy

This procedure, which removes half of the brain's cortex, or outer layer, is used only for children who have Rasmussen's encephalitis or other severe damage to one brain hemisphere and who also have seizures that do not respond well to medication. While this type of surgery is very radical and is performed only as a last resort, children often recover very well from the procedure, and their seizures usually are greatly reduced or may cease altogether. With intense rehabilitation, they often recover nearly normal abilities. Since the chance of a full recovery is best in young children, hemispherectomy should be performed as early in a child's life as possible. It is almost never performed in children older than 13.

Devices

The vagus nerve stimulator was approved by the U.S. Food and Drug Administration (FDA) in 1997 for use in people with seizures that are not well-controlled by medication. The vagus nerve stimulator is a battery-powered device that is surgically implanted under the skin of the chest, much like a pacemaker, and is attached to the vagus nerve in the lower neck. This device delivers short bursts of electrical energy to the brain via the vagus nerve. On average, this stimulation reduces seizures by about 20-40 percent. Patients usually cannot stop taking epilepsy medication because of the stimulator, but they often experience fewer seizures and they may be able to reduce the dose of their medication. Side effects of the vagus nerve stimulator are generally mild, but may include ear pain, a sore throat, or nausea. Adjusting the amount of stimulation can usually eliminate these side effects. The batteries in the vagus nerve stimulator need to be replaced about once every 5 years; this requires a minor operation that can usually be performed as an outpatient procedure.

Several new devices may become available for epilepsy in the future. Researchers are studying whether transcranial magnetic stimulation, a procedure which uses a strong magnet held outside the head to influence brain activity, may reduce seizures. They also hope to develop implantable devices that can deliver drugs to specific parts of the brain.

Diet

Studies have shown that, in some cases, children may experience fewer seizures if they maintain a strict diet rich in fats and low in carbohydrates. This unusual diet, called the ketogenic diet, causes the body to break down fats instead of carbohydrates to survive. This condition is called ketosis. One study of 150 children whose seizures were poorly controlled by medication found that about one-fourth of the children had a 90 percent or better decrease in seizures with the ketogenic diet, and another half of the group had a 50 percent or better decrease in their seizures. Moreover, some children can discontinue the ketogenic diet after several years and remain seizure-free. The ketogenic diet is not easy to maintain, as it requires strict adherence to an unusual and limited range of foods. Possible side effects include retarded growth due to nutritional deficiency and a buildup of uric acid in the blood, which can lead to kidney stones. People who try the ketogenic diet should seek the guidance of a dietician to ensure that it does not lead to serious nutritional deficiency.

Researchers are not sure how ketosis inhibits seizures. One study showed that a byproduct of ketosis called beta-hydroxybutyrate (BHB) inhibits seizures in animals. If BHB also works in humans, researchers may eventually be able to develop drugs that mimic the seizure-inhibiting effects of the ketogenic diet.

Other Treatment Strategies

Researchers are studying whether biofeedback—a strategy in which individuals learn to control their own brain waves—may be useful in controlling seizures. However, this type of therapy is controversial and most studies have shown discouraging results. Taking large doses of vitamins generally does not help a person's seizures and may even be harmful in some cases. However, a good diet and some vitamin supplements, particularly folic acid, may help reduce some birth defects and medication-related nutritional deficiencies. Use of non-vitamin supplements such as melatonin is controversial and can be risky. One study showed that melatonin may reduce seizures in some children, while another found that the risk of seizures increased measurably with melatonin. Most non-vitamin supplements such as those found in health food stores are not regulated by the FDA, so their true effects and their interactions with other drugs are largely unknown.

How Does Epilepsy Affect Daily Life?

Most people with epilepsy lead outwardly normal lives. Approximately 80 percent can be significantly helped by modern therapies, and some may go months or years between seizures. However, epilepsy can and does affect daily life for people with epilepsy, their families, and their friends. People with severe seizures that resist treatment have, on average, a shorter life expectancy and an increased risk of cognitive impairment, particularly if the seizures developed in early childhood. These impairments may be related to the underlying conditions that cause epilepsy or to epilepsy treatment rather than the epilepsy itself.

Behavior and Emotions

It is not uncommon for people with epilepsy, especially children, to develop behavioral and emotional problems. Sometimes these problems are caused by embarrassment or frustration associated with epilepsy. Other problems may result from bullying, teasing, or avoidance in school and other social settings. In children, these problems can be minimized if parents encourage a positive outlook and independence, do not reward negative behavior with unusual amounts of attention, and try to stay attuned to their child's needs and feelings. Families must learn to accept and live with the seizures without blaming or resenting the affected person. Counseling services can help families cope with epilepsy in a positive manner. Epilepsy support groups also can help by providing a way for people with epilepsy and their family members to share their experiences, frustrations, and tips for coping with the disorder.

People with epilepsy have an increased risk of poor self-esteem, depression, and suicide. These problems may be a reaction to a lack of understanding or discomfort about epilepsy that may result in cruelty or avoidance by other people. Many people with epilepsy also live with an ever-present fear that they will have another seizure.

Driving and Recreation

For many people with epilepsy, the risk of seizures restricts their independence, in particular the ability to drive. Most states and the District of Columbia will not issue a driver's license to someone with epilepsy unless the person can document that they have gone a specific amount of time without a seizure (the waiting period varies from a few months to several years). Some states make exceptions for this policy when seizures don't impair consciousness, occur only during sleep, or have long auras or other warning signs that allow the person to avoid driving when a seizure is likely to occur. Studies show that the risk of having a seizure-related accident decreases as the length of time since the last seizure increases. One study found that the risk of having a seizure-related motor vehicle accident is 93 percent less in people who wait at least 1 year after their last seizure before driving, compared to people who wait for shorter intervals.

The risk of seizures also restricts people's recreational choices. For instance, people with epilepsy should not participate in sports such as skydiving or motor racing where a moment's inattention could lead to injury. Other activities, such as swimming and sailing, should be done only with precautions and/or supervision. However, jogging, football, and many other sports are reasonably safe for a person with epilepsy. Studies to date have not shown any increase in seizures due to sports, although these studies have not focused on any activity in particular. There is some evidence that regular exercise may even improve seizure control in some people. Sports are often such a positive factor in life that it is best for the person to participate, although the person with epilepsy and the coach or other leader should take appropriate safety precautions. It is important to take steps to avoid potential sports-related problems such as dehydration, overexertion, and hypoglycemia, as these problems can increase the risk of seizures.

Education and Employment

By law, people with epilepsy or other handicaps in the United States cannot be denied employment or access to any educational, recreational, or other activity because of their seizures. However, one survey showed that only about 56 percent of people with epilepsy finish high school and about 15 percent finish college — rates much lower than those for the general population. The same survey found that about 25 percent of working-age people with epilepsy are unemployed. These numbers indicate that significant barriers still exist for people with epilepsy in school and work. Restrictions on driving limit the employment opportunities for many people with epilepsy, and many find it difficult to face the misunderstandings and social pressures they encounter in public situations. Antiepileptic drugs also may cause side effects that interfere with concentration and memory. Children with epilepsy may need extra time to complete schoolwork, and they sometimes may need to have instructions or other information repeated for them. Teachers should be told what to do if a child in their classroom has a seizure, and parents should work with the school system to find reasonable ways to accommodate any special needs their child may have.

Pregnancy and Motherhood

Women with epilepsy are often concerned about whether they can become pregnant and have a healthy child. This is usually possible. While some seizure medications and some types of epilepsy may reduce a person's interest in sexual activity, most people with epilepsy can become pregnant. Moreover, women with epilepsy have a 90 percent or better chance of having a normal, healthy baby, and the risk of birth defects is only about 4-6 percent. The risk that children of parents with epilepsy will develop epilepsy themselves is only about 5 percent unless the parent has a clearly hereditary form of the disorder. Parents who are worried that their epilepsy may be hereditary may wish to consult a genetic counselor to determine what the risk might be. Amniocentesis and high-level ultrasound can be performed during pregnancy to ensure that the baby is developing normally, and a procedure called a maternal serum alpha-fetoprotein test can be used for prenatal diagnosis of many conditions if a problem is suspected.

There are several precautions women can take before and during pregnancy to reduce the risks associated with pregnancy and delivery. Women who are thinking about becoming pregnant should talk with their doctors to learn any special risks associated with their epilepsy and the medications they may be taking. Some seizure medications, particularly valproate, trimethadione, and phenytoin, are known to increase the risk of having a child with birth defects such as cleft palate, heart problems, or finger and toe defects. For this reason, a woman's doctor may advise switching to other medications during pregnancy. Whenever possible, a woman should allow her doctor enough time to properly change medications, including phasing in the new medications and checking to determine when blood levels are stabilized, before she tries to become pregnant. Women should also begin prenatal vitamin supplements — especially with folic acid, which may reduce the risk of some birth defects — well before pregnancy. Women who discover that they are pregnant but have not already spoken with their doctor about ways to reduce the risks should do so as soon as possible. However, they should continue taking seizure medication as prescribed until that time to avoid preventable seizures. Seizures during pregnancy can harm the developing baby or lead to miscarriage, particularly if the seizures are severe. Nevertheless, many women who have seizures during pregnancy have normal, healthy babies.

Women with epilepsy sometimes experience a change in their seizure frequency during pregnancy, even if they do not change medications. About 25 to 40 percent of women have an increase in their seizure frequency while they are pregnant, while other women may have fewer seizures during pregnancy. The frequency of seizures during pregnancy may be influenced by a variety of factors, including the woman's increased blood volume during pregnancy, which can dilute the effect of medication. Women should have their blood levels of seizure medications monitored closely during and after pregnancy, and the medication dosage should be adjusted accordingly.

Pregnant women with epilepsy should take prenatal vitamins and get plenty of sleep to avoid seizures caused by sleep deprivation. They also should take vitamin K supplements after 34 weeks of pregnancy to reduce the risk of a blood-clotting disorder in infants called neonatal coagulopathy that can result from fetal exposure to epilepsy medications. Finally, they should get good prenatal care, avoid tobacco, caffeine, alcohol, and illegal drugs, and try to avoid stress.

Labor and delivery usually proceed normally for women with epilepsy, although there is a slightly increased risk of hemorrhage, eclampsia, premature labor, and cesarean section. Doctors can administer antiepileptic drugs intravenously and monitor blood levels of anticonvulsant medication during labor to reduce the risk that the labor will trigger a seizure. Babies sometimes have symptoms of withdrawal from the mother's seizure medication after they are born, but these problems wear off in a few weeks or months and usually do not cause serious or long-term effects. A mother's blood levels of anticonvulsant medication should be checked frequently after delivery as medication often needs to be decreased.

Epilepsy medications need not influence a woman's decision about breast-feeding her baby. Only minor amounts of epilepsy medications are secreted in breast milk; usually not enough to harm the baby and much less than the baby was exposed to in the womb. On rare occasions, the baby may become excessively drowsy or feed poorly, and these problems should be closely monitored. However, experts believe the benefits of breast-feeding outweigh the risks except in rare circumstances.

To increase doctors' understanding of how different epilepsy medications affect pregnancy and the chances of having a healthy baby, Massachusetts General Hospital has begun a nationwide registry for women who take antiepileptic drugs while pregnant. Women who enroll in this program are given educational materials on pre-conception planning and perinatal care and are asked to provide information about the health of their children (this information is kept confidential). Women and physicians can contact this registry by calling 1-888-233-2334 or 617-726-7739 (fax: 617-724-8307).

Women with epilepsy should be aware that some epilepsy medications can interfere with the effectiveness of oral contraceptives. Women who wish to use oral contraceptives to prevent pregnancy should discuss this with their doctors, who may be able to prescribe a different kind of antiepileptic medication or suggest other ways of avoiding an unplanned pregnancy.

Are There Special Risks Associated with Epilepsy?

Although most people with epilepsy lead full, active lives, they are at special risk for two life-threatening conditions: status epilepticus and sudden unexplained death.

Status Epilepticus

Status epilepticus is a severe, life-threatening condition in which a person either has prolonged seizures or does not fully regain consciousness between seizures. The amount of time in a prolonged seizure that must pass before a person should be diagnosed with status epilepticus is a subject of debate. Many doctors now diagnose status epilepticus if a person has been in a prolonged seizure for 5 minutes. However, other doctors use more conservative definitions of this condition and may not diagnose status epilepticus unless the person has had a prolonged seizure of 10 minutes or even 30 minutes.

Status epilepticus affects about 195,000 people each year in the United States and results in about 42,000 deaths. While people with epilepsy are at an increased risk for status epilepticus, about 60 percent of people who develop this condition have no previous seizure history. These cases often result from tumors, trauma, or other problems that affect the brain and may themselves be life-threatening.

While most seizures do not require emergency medical treatment, someone with a prolonged seizure lasting more than 5 minutes may be in status epilepticus and should be taken to an emergency room immediately. It is important to treat a person with status epilepticus as soon as possible. One study showed that 80 percent of people in status epilepticus who received medication within 30 minutes of seizure onset eventually stopped having seizures, whereas only 40 percent recovered if 2 hours had passed before they received medication. Doctors in a hospital setting can treat status epilepticus with several different drugs and can undertake emergency life-saving measures, such as administering oxygen, if necessary.

People in status epilepticus do not always have severe convulsive seizures. Instead, they may have repeated or prolonged nonconvulsive seizures. This type of status epilepticus may appear as a sustained episode of confusion or agitation in someone who does not ordinarily have that kind of mental impairment. While this type of episode may not seem as severe as convulsive status epilepticus, it should still be treated as an emergency.

Sudden Unexplained Death

For reasons that are poorly understood, people with epilepsy have an increased risk of dying suddenly for no discernible reason. This condition, called sudden unexplained death, can occur in people without epilepsy, but epilepsy increases the risk about two-fold. Researchers are still unsure why sudden unexplained death occurs. One study suggested that use of more than two anticonvulsant drugs may be a risk factor. However, it is not clear whether the use of multiple drugs causes the sudden death, or whether people who use multiple anticonvulsants have a greater risk of death because they have more severe types of epilepsy.

What Research Is Being Done on Epilepsy?

While research has led to many advances in understanding and treating epilepsy, there are many unanswered questions about how and why seizures develop, how they can best be treated or prevented, and how they influence other brain activity and brain development. Researchers, many of whom are supported by the National Institute of Neurological Disorders and Stroke (NINDS), are studying all of these questions. They also are working to identify and test new drugs and other treatments for epilepsy and to learn how those treatments affect brain activity and development. NINDS' Epilepsy Therapeutics Research Program studies potential antiepileptic drugs with the goal of enhancing treatment for epilepsy. Since it began in 1975, this program has screened more than 22,000 compounds for their potential as antiepileptic drugs and has contributed to the development of five drugs that are now approved for use in the United States as well as others that are still being developed or tested.

Scientists continue to study how excitatory and inhibitory neurotransmitters interact with brain cells to control nerve firing. They can apply different chemicals to cultures of neurons in laboratory dishes to study how those chemicals influence neuronal activity. They also are studying how glia and other non-neuronal cells in the brain contribute to seizures. This research may lead to new drugs and other new ways of treating seizures.

Researchers also are working to identify genes that may influence epilepsy in some way. Identifying these genes can reveal the underlying chemical processes that influence epilepsy and point to new ways of preventing or treating this disorder. Researchers also can study rats and mice that have missing or abnormal copies of certain genes to determine how these genes affect normal brain development and resistance to damage from disease and other environmental factors. Researchers may soon be able to use devices called gene chips to determine each person's genetic makeup or to learn which genes are active. This information may allow doctors to prevent epilepsy or to predict which treatments will be most beneficial.

Doctors are now experimenting with several new types of therapies for epilepsy. In one preliminary clinical trial, doctors have begun transplanting fetal pig neurons that produce GABA into the brains of patients to learn whether the cell transplants can help control seizures. Preliminary research suggests that stem cell transplants also may prove beneficial for treating epilepsy. Research showing that the brain undergoes subtle changes prior to a seizure has led to a prototype device that may be able to predict seizures up to 3 minutes before they begin. If this device works, it could greatly reduce the risk of injury from seizures by allowing people to move to a safe area before their seizures start. This type of device also may be hooked up to a treatment pump or other device that will automatically deliver an antiepileptic drug or an electric impulse to forestall the seizures.

Researchers are continually improving MRI and other brain scans. Pre-surgical brain imaging can guide doctors to abnormal brain tissue and away from essential parts of the brain. Researchers also are using brain scans such as magnetoencephalograms (MEG) and magnetic resonance spectroscopy (MRS) to identify and study subtle problems in the brain that cannot otherwise be detected. Their findings may lead to a better understanding of epilepsy and how it can be treated.

How Can I Help Research on Epilepsy?

There are many ways that people with epilepsy and their families can help with research on this disorder. Pregnant women with epilepsy who are taking antiepileptic drugs can help researchers learn how these drugs affect unborn children by participating in the Antiepileptic Drug Pregnancy Registry, which is maintained by the Genetics and Teratology Unit of Massachusetts General Hospital (see section on Pregnancy and Motherhood). People with epilepsy that may be hereditary can aid research by participating in the Epilepsy Gene Discovery Project, which is supported by the Epilepsy Foundation. This project helps to educate people with epilepsy about new genetic research on the disorder and enlists families with hereditary epilepsy for participation in gene research. People who enroll in this project are asked to create a family tree showing which people in their family have or have had epilepsy. Researchers then examine this information to determine if the epilepsy is in fact hereditary, and they may invite participants to enroll in genetic research studies. In many cases, identifying the gene defect responsible for epilepsy in an individual family leads researchers to new clues about how epilepsy develops. It also can provide opportunities for early diagnosis and genetic screening of individuals in the family.

People with epilepsy can help researchers test new medications, surgical techniques, and other treatments by enrolling in clinical trials. Information on clinical trials can be obtained from the NINDS as well as many private pharmaceutical and biotech companies, universities, and other organizations. A person who wishes to participate in a clinical trial must ask his or her regular physician to refer him or her to the doctor in charge of that trial and to forward all necessary medical records. While experimental therapies may benefit those who participate in clinical trials, patients and their families should remember that all clinical trials also involve some risks. Therapies being tested in clinical trials may not work, and in some cases doctors may not yet be certain that the therapies are safe. Patients should be certain they understand the risks before agreeing to participate in a clinical trial.

NINDS supports a number of Epilepsy Research Centers that perform a broad spectrum of clinical research on epilepsy. Some of the studies require patient volunteers. A list of these centers is available from the NIH Neurological Institute, which can be reached at the address and phone number found on the Information Resources card in the back pocket of this brochure.

Patients and their families also can help epilepsy research by donating their brain to a brain bank after death. Brain banks supply researchers with tissue they can use to study epilepsy and other disorders. Below are some brain banks that accept tissue from patients with epilepsy:

Brain and Tissue Bank for Neurological Disorders
University of Maryland, Baltimore
Dr. Ron Zielke
Director
800-847-1539
www.som1.umaryland.edu/BTBank/

Brain and Tissue Bank for Developmental Disorders
University of Miami
Dr. Carol Petito
Director
800-59Brain (592-7246)
E-mail: btbcoord@med.Miami.edu
Fax: 305-243-6970
Tissue from children only.

Brain Endowment Bank
University of Miami
Dr. Deborah Mash
Director
800-UMBrain (862-7246)
FAX: 305-243-3649
Tissue from adults only.

National Disease Research Interchange
1880 JFK Boulevard, 6th Floor
Philadelphia, Pennsylvania 19103
215-557-7361
800-222-NDRI (6374)

National Neurological Research Specimen Bank

VAMC (W127A)-West Los Angeles
11301 Wilshire Boulevard
Los Angeles, California 90073
310-268-3536
24-hour pager: 310-636-5199

What to Do If You See Someone Having a Seizure

If you see someone having a seizure with convulsions and/or loss of consciousness, here's how you can help:

- Roll the person on his or her side to prevent choking on any fluids or vomit.

- Cushion the person's head.

- Loosen any tight clothing around the neck.

- Keep the person's airway open. If necessary, grip the person's jaw gently and tilt his or her head back.

- Do NOT restrict the person from moving unless he or she is in danger.

- Do NOT put anything into the person's mouth, not even medicine or liquid. These can cause choking or damage to the person's jaw, tongue, or teeth. Contrary to widespread belief, people cannot swallow their tongues during a seizure or any other time.

- Remove any sharp or solid objects that the person might hit during the seizure.

- Note how long the seizure lasts and what symptoms occurred so you can tell a doctor or emergency personnel if necessary.

- Stay with the person until the seizure ends.

Call 911 if:

- The person is pregnant or has diabetes.

- The seizure happened in water.

- The seizure lasts longer than 5 minutes.

- The person does not begin breathing again and return to consciousness after the seizure stops.

- Another seizure starts before the person regains consciousness.

- The person injures himself or herself during the seizure.

- This is a first seizure or you think it might be. If in doubt, check to see if the person has a medical identification card or jewelry stating that he or she has epilepsy or a seizure disorder.

After the seizure ends, the person will probably be groggy and tired. He or she also may have a headache and be confused or embarrassed. Be patient with the person and try to help him or her find a place to rest if he or she is tired or doesn't feel well. If necessary, offer to call a taxi, a friend, or a relative to help the person get home safely.

If you see someone having a non-convulsive seizure, remember that the person's behavior is not intentional. The person may wander aimlessly or make alarming or unusual gestures. You can help by following these guidelines:

- Remove any dangerous objects from the area around the person or in his or her path.

- Don't try to stop the person from wandering unless he or she is in danger.

- Don't shake the person or shout.

- Stay with the person until he or she is completely alert.

Conclusion

Many people with epilepsy lead productive and outwardly normal lives. Many medical and research advances in the past two decades have led to a better understanding of epilepsy and seizures than ever before. Advanced brain scans and other techniques allow greater accuracy in diagnosing epilepsy and determining when a patient may be helped by surgery. More than 20 different medications and a variety of surgical techniques are now available and provide good control of seizures for most people with epilepsy. Other treatment options include the ketogenic diet and the first implantable device, the vagus nerve stimulator. Research on the underlying causes of epilepsy, including identification of genes for some forms of epilepsy and febrile seizures, has led to a greatly improved understanding of epilepsy that may lead to more effective treatments or even new ways of preventing epilepsy in the future.

Information Resources

The National Institute of Neurological Disorders and Stroke, a component of the National Institutes of Health, is the leading Federal supporter of research on disorders of the brain and nervous system. The Institute also sponsors an active public information program with staff who can answer questions about diagnosis and research related to seizures and epilepsy. For information on seizures or other neurological disorders, contact the Institute's Brain Resources and Information Network (BRAIN) at:

BRAIN
P.O. Box 5801
Bethesda, Maryland 20824
800-352-9424
www.ninds.nih.gov

Private voluntary organizations that provide information on treatment, diagnosis, and services include the following:

American Epilepsy Society
342 North Main Street
West Hartford, Connecticut 06117
860-586-7505
www.aesnet.org
The American Epilepsy Society, one of the oldest neurological professional organizations in the country, promotes research and education for professionals interested in seizure disorders and epilepsy. Membership consists of clinicians, scientists investigating basic and clinical aspects of epilepsy, and other professionals interested in both pediatric and adult seizure disorders. The Society develops resources and collaborative relationships worldwide to advance patient care and to support efforts leading to the prevention, treatment, and cure of epilepsy. It also holds an annual scientific meeting that attracts more than 3,500 professionals.

Citizens United for Research in Epilepsy (CURE)
505 North Lake Shore Drive, #4605
Chicago, Illinois 60611
312-923-9117
312-923-9118 (fax)
CUReepi@aol.com
www.CUREepilepsy.org

CURE is a global grassroots organization dedicated to finding a cure for pediatric intractable epilepsy. CURE works to stimulate innovative epilepsy research through private funding sources and by publishing the long overlooked need for a cure for this disease.

Epilepsy Foundation
4351 Garden City Drive
Suite 500
Landover, Maryland 20785
301-459-3700
800-332-1000
301-577-2684 (fax)
postmaster@efa.org
www.epilepsyfoundation.org
The Epilepsy Foundation is a national voluntary health agency that works for people affected by seizures through research, education, advocacy, and service. Its goals are the prevention and cure of seizure disorders, the alleviation of their effects, and the promotion of independence and optimal quality of life for people who have these disorders. Epilepsy Foundation affiliates serve people with epilepsy and their families in more than 100 communities throughout the United States.

National Association of Epilepsy Centers
5775 Wayzata Boulevard
Suite 200
Minneapolis, Minnesota 55416
952-525-4526
The goals of this Association, which includes the majority of specialized epilepsy centers in the U.S., are to provide information about the care of patients with epilepsy to the appropriate government and industry officials; to exchange information among its members; and to participate in developing standards for programs providing services.

Epilepsy Institute
257 Park Avenue South
New York, NY 10010
212-677-8550
212-677-5825 (fax)
website@epilepsyinstitute.org
www.epilepsyinstitute.org
A non-profit organization that provides comprehensive social services and resources for people with epilepsy and their families.

National Organization for Rare Disorders (NORD)
P.O. Box 8923
100 Route 37
New Fairfield, Connecticut 06812-8923
203-746-6518
800-999-NORD (6673)
203-746-6481 (fax)
orphan@rarediseases.org
www.rarediseases.org
The National Organization for Rare Disorders (NORD), a federation of voluntary health organizations dedicated to helping people with rare "orphan"diseases, is committed to the identification, treatment, and cure of rare disorders through programs of education, advocacy, research, and service.

For information on prescription medicines, contact:

National Council on Patient Information and Education
4915 St. Elmo Avenue
Suite 505
Bethesda, Maryland 20814
301-656-8565
301-656-4464 (fax)
ncpie@erols.com
www.talkaboutrx.org
The National Council on Patient Information and Education is a coalition of organizations committed to providing patients, consumers, and caregivers with useful and appropriate medicine information.

Pregnant women with epilepsy can help researchers learn how epilepsy drugs affect unborn children by participating in the following program:

Antiepileptic Drug Pregnancy Registry
Massachusetts General Hospital
Genetics and Teratology Unit
55 Fruit Street
Boston, Massachusetts 02114
888-233-2334
http://www.aedpregnancyregistry.org/

Other support organizations include:

Family Caregiver Alliance
690 Market Street, Suite 600
San Francisco, California 94104
415-434-3388
800-445-8106
415-434-3508 (fax)
info@caregiver.org
www.caregiver.org
Services offered by the Family Caregiver Alliance include specialized information and assistance, consultation on long-term care planning, service linkage and arrangement, legal and financial consultation, respite services, counseling, and education.

National Family Caregivers Association
10400 Connecticut Avenue
Suite 500
Kensington, Maryland 20895
301-942-6430
800-896-365
301-942-2302 (fax)
info@nfacares.org
www.nfcacares.org
Through its services in the areas of education and information, support and validation, public awareness, and advocacy, the National Family Caregivers Association strives to improve caregivers' quality of life.

ONLINE GLOSSARIES

The Internet provides access to a number of free-to-use medical dictionaries and glossaries. The National Library of Medicine has compiled the following list of online dictionaries:

- ADAM Medical Encyclopedia (A.D.A.M., Inc.), comprehensive medical reference: **http://www.nlm.nih.gov/medlineplus/encyclopedia.html**

- MedicineNet.com Medical Dictionary (MedicineNet, Inc.): **http://www.medterms.com/Script/Main/hp.asp**

- Merriam-Webster Medical Dictionary (Inteli-Health, Inc.): **http://www.intelihealth.com/IH/**

- Multilingual Glossary of Technical and Popular Medical Terms in Eight European Languages (European Commission) - Danish, Dutch, English, French, German, Italian, Portuguese, and Spanish: **http://allserv.rug.ac.be/~rvdstich/eugloss/welcome.html**

- On-line Medical Dictionary (CancerWEB): **http://www.graylab.ac.uk/omd/**

- Technology Glossary (National Library of Medicine) - Health Care Technology: **http://www.nlm.nih.gov/nichsr/ta101/ta10108.htm**

- Terms and Definitions (Office of Rare Diseases): **http://rarediseases.info.nih.gov/ord/glossary_a-e.html**

Beyond these, MEDLINEplus contains a very user-friendly encyclopedia covering every aspect of medicine (licensed from A.D.A.M., Inc.). The ADAM Medical Encyclopedia can be accessed via the following Web site address: **http://www.nlm.nih.gov/medlineplus/encyclopedia.html**. ADAM is also available on commercial Web sites such as Web MD (**http://my.webmd.com/adam/asset/adam_disease_articles/a_to_z/a**) and drkoop.com (**http://www.drkoop.com/**). Topics of interest can be researched by using keywords before continuing elsewhere, as these basic definitions and concepts will be useful in more advanced areas of research. You may choose to print various pages specifically relating to infantile spasms and keep them on file.

Online Dictionary Directories

The following are additional online directories compiled by the National Library of Medicine, including a number of specialized medical dictionaries and glossaries:

- Medical Dictionaries: Medical & Biological (World Health Organization): **http://www.who.int/hlt/virtuallibrary/English/diction.htm#Medical**

- MEL-Michigan Electronic Library List of Online Health and Medical Dictionaries (Michigan Electronic Library): **http://mel.lib.mi.us/health/health-dictionaries.html**

- Patient Education: Glossaries (DMOZ Open Directory Project): **http://dmoz.org/Health/Education/Patient_Education/Glossaries/**

- Web of Online Dictionaries (Bucknell University): **http://www.yourdictionary.com/diction5.html#medicine**

INFANTILE SPASMS GLOSSARY

The following is a complete glossary of terms used in this sourcebook. The definitions are derived from official public sources including the National Institutes of Health [NIH] and the European Union [EU]. After this glossary, we list a number of additional hardbound and electronic glossaries and dictionaries that you may wish to consult.

Agenesis: Lack of complete or normal development; congenital absence of an organ or part. [NIH]

Airway: A device for securing unobstructed passage of air into and out of the lungs during general anesthesia. [NIH]

Anticonvulsive: An agent that prevents or relieves convulsions. [NIH]

Apnea: Cessation of breathing. [NIH]

Asynchronous: Pacing mode where only one timing interval exists, that between the stimuli. While the duration of this interval may be varied, it is not modified by any sensed event once set. As no sensing occurs, the upper and lower rate intervals are the same as the pacema. [NIH]

Branch: Most commonly used for branches of nerves, but applied also to other structures. [NIH]

Breakdown: A physical, metal, or nervous collapse. [NIH]

Compassionate: A process for providing experimental drugs to very sick patients who have no treatment options. [NIH]

Consultation: A deliberation between two or more physicians concerning the diagnosis and the proper method of treatment in a case. [NIH]

Consumption: Pulmonary tuberculosis. [NIH]

Contraindications: Any factor or sign that it is unwise to pursue a certain kind of action or treatment, e. g. giving a general anesthetic to a person with pneumonia. [NIH]

Cortisol: A steroid hormone secreted by the adrenal cortex as part of the body's response to stress. [NIH]

Crichton: Twitching of the outer corners of the eyes and the lips indicating syphilitic meningoencephalitis. [NIH]

Deletion: A genetic rearrangement through loss of segments of DNA (chromosomes), bringing sequences, which are normally separated, into close proximity. [NIH]

Discrete: Made up of separate parts or characterized by lesions which do not become blended; not running together; separate. [NIH]

Discrimination: The act of qualitative and/or quantitative differentiation between two or more stimuli. [NIH]

EEG: A graphic recording of the changes in electrical potential associated with the activity of the cerebral cortex made with the electroencephalogram. [NIH]

Electrode: Component of the pacing system which is at the distal end of the lead. It is the interface with living cardiac tissue across which the stimulus is transmitted. [NIH]

Endorphin: Opioid peptides derived from beta-lipotropin. Endorphin is the most potent naturally occurring analgesic agent. It is present in pituitary, brain, and peripheral tissues. [NIH]

Epilepsia: An illusional seizure consisting of a rather sudden alteration of the patient's perceptions, indicative of a lesion in the temporal lobes. [NIH]

Epilepticus: Repeated and prolonged epileptic seizures without recovery of consciousness between attacks. [NIH]

Excitability: Property of a cardiac cell whereby, when the cell is depolarized to a critical level (called threshold), the membrane becomes permeable and a regenerative inward current causes an action potential. [NIH]

Excitotoxicity: Excessive exposure to glutamate or related compounds can kill brain neurons, presumably by overstimulating them. [NIH]

Fatigue: The feeling of weariness of mind and body. [NIH]

Fetoprotein: Transabdominal aspiration of fluid from the amniotic sac with a view to detecting increases of alpha-fetoprotein in maternal blood during pregnancy, as this is an important indicator of open neural tube defects in the fetus. [NIH]

Fold: A plication or doubling of various parts of the body. [NIH]

Fossa: A cavity, depression, or pit. [NIH]

Genetics: The biological science that deals with the phenomena and mechanisms of heredity. [NIH]

Gould: Turning of the head downward in walking to bring the image of the ground on the functioning position of the retina, in destructive disease of the peripheral retina. [NIH]

Growth: The progressive development of a living being or part of an organism from its earliest stage to maturity. [NIH]

Handicap: A handicap occurs as a result of disability, but disability does not always constitute a handicap. A handicap may be said to exist when a disability causes a substantial and continuing reduction in a person's capacity to function socially and vocationally. [NIH]

Harmony: Attribute of a product which gives rise to an overall pleasant sensation. This sensation is produced by the perception of the product components as olfactory, gustatory, tactile and kinaesthetic stimuli because they are present in suitable concentration ratios. [NIH]

Hereditary: Of, relating to, or denoting factors that can be transmitted genetically from one generation to another. [NIH]

HLA: A glycoprotein found on the surface of all human leucocytes. The HLA region of chromosome 6 produces four such glycoproteins-A, B, C and D. [NIH]

Homeobox: Distinctive sequence of DNA bases. [NIH]

Host: Any animal that receives a transplanted graft. [NIH]

Impairment: In the context of health experience, an impairment is any loss or abnormality of psychological, physiological, or anatomical structure or function. [NIH]

Infancy: The period of complete dependency prior to the acquisition of competence in walking, talking, and self-feeding. [NIH]

Infections: The illnesses caused by an organism that usually does not cause disease in a person with a normal immune system. [NIH]

Insight: The capacity to understand one's own motives, to be aware of one's own psychodynamics, to appreciate the meaning of symbolic behavior. [NIH]

Isoenzyme: Different forms of an enzyme, usually occurring in different tissues. The isoenzymes of a particular enzyme catalyze the same reaction but they differ in some of their properties. [NIH]

Jefferson: A fracture produced by a compressive downward force that is transmitted evenly through occipital condyles to superior articular surfaces of the lateral masses of C1. [NIH]

Joint: The point of contact between elements of an animal skeleton with the parts that surround and support it. [NIH]

Linkage: The tendency of two or more genes in the same chromosome to remain together from one generation to the next more frequently than expected according to the law of independent assortment. [NIH]

Medial: Lying near the midsaggital plane of the body; opposed to lateral. [NIH]

Migration: The systematic movement of genes between populations of the same species, geographic race, or variety. [NIH]

Miscarriage: Spontaneous expulsion of the products of pregnancy before the middle of the second trimester. [NIH]

Modeling: A treatment procedure whereby the therapist presents the target behavior which the learner is to imitate and make part of his repertoire. [NIH]

Monoamine: Enzyme that breaks down dopamine in the astrocytes and microglia. [NIH]

Morphological: Relating to the configuration or the structure of live organs. [NIH]

Narcolepsy: A condition of unknown cause characterized by a periodic uncontrollable tendency to fall asleep. [NIH]

Need: A state of tension or dissatisfaction felt by an individual that impels him to action toward a goal he believes will satisfy the impulse. [NIH]

Nerve: A cordlike structure of nervous tissue that connects parts of the nervous system with other tissues of the body and conveys nervous impulses to, or away from, these tissues. [NIH]

Networks: Pertaining to a nerve or to the nerves, a meshlike structure of interlocking fibers or strands. [NIH]

Nuclei: A body of specialized protoplasm found in nearly all cells and containing the chromosomes. [NIH]

Outpatient: A patient who is not an inmate of a hospital but receives diagnosis or treatment in a clinic or dispensary connected with the hospital. [NIH]

Palsy: Disease of the peripheral nervous system occurring usually after many years of increased lead absorption. [NIH]

Papilloma: A benign epithelial neoplasm which may arise from the skin, mucous membranes or glandular ducts. [NIH]

Phenotypes: An organism as observed, i. e. as judged by its visually perceptible characters resulting from the interaction of its genotype with the environment. [NIH]

Potassium: It is essential to the ability of muscle cells to contract. [NIH]

Protocol: The detailed plan for a clinical trial that states the trial's rationale, purpose, drug or vaccine dosages, length of study, routes of administration, who may participate, and other aspects of trial design. [NIH]

Race: A population within a species which exhibits general similarities within itself, but is both discontinuous and distinct from other populations of that species, though not sufficiently so as to achieve the status of a taxon. [NIH]

Restoration: Broad term applied to any inlay, crown, bridge or complete denture which restores or replaces loss of teeth or oral tissues. [NIH]

Schizophrenia: A mental disorder characterized by a special type of disintegration of the personality. [NIH]

Segmental: Describing or pertaining to a structure which is repeated in similar form in successive segments of an organism, or which is undergoing segmentation. [NIH]

Specialist: In medicine, one who concentrates on 1 special branch of medical science. [NIH]

Spectroscopic: The recognition of elements through their emission spectra. [NIH]

Sperm: The fecundating fluid of the male. [NIH]

Temporal: One of the two irregular bones forming part of the lateral surfaces and base of the skull, and containing the organs of hearing. [NIH]

Thalamic: Cell that reaches the lateral nucleus of amygdala. [NIH]

Therapeutics: The branch of medicine which is concerned with the treatment of diseases, palliative or curative. [NIH]

Threshold: For a specified sensory modality (e. g. light, sound, vibration), the lowest level (absolute threshold) or smallest difference (difference threshold, difference limen) or intensity of the stimulus discernible in prescribed conditions of stimulation. [NIH]

Translocation: The movement of material in solution inside the body of the plant. [NIH]

Trauma: Any injury, wound, or shock, must frequently physical or structural shock, producing a disturbance. [NIH]

Tuberous Sclerosis: A rare congenital disease in which the essential pathology is the appearance of multiple tumors in the cerebrum and in other organs, such as the heart or kidneys. [NIH]

Ulcer: A localized necrotic lesion of the skin or a mucous surface. [NIH]

Unconscious: Experience which was once conscious, but was subsequently rejected, as the "personal unconscious". [NIH]

Vivo: Outside of or removed from the body of a living organism. [NIH]

Womb: A hollow, thick-walled, muscular organ in which the impregnated ovum is developed into a child. [NIH]

Wound: Any interruption, by violence or by surgery, in the continuity of the external surface of the body or of the surface of any internal organ. [NIH]

General Dictionaries and Glossaries

While the above glossary is essentially complete, the dictionaries listed here cover virtually all aspects of medicine, from basic words and phrases to more advanced terms (sorted alphabetically by title; hyperlinks provide rankings, information and reviews at Amazon.com):

- **Dictionary of Medical Acronymns & Abbreviations** by Stanley Jablonski (Editor), Paperback, 4th edition (2001), Lippincott Williams & Wilkins

Publishers, ISBN: 1560534605,
http://www.amazon.com/exec/obidos/ASIN/1560534605/icongroupinter
na

- **Dictionary of Medical Terms : For the Nonmedical Person (Dictionary of Medical Terms for the Nonmedical Person, Ed 4)** by Mikel A. Rothenberg, M.D, et al, Paperback - 544 pages, 4th edition (2000), Barrons Educational Series, ISBN: 0764112015,
http://www.amazon.com/exec/obidos/ASIN/0764112015/icongroupinter
na

- **A Dictionary of the History of Medicine** by A. Sebastian, CD-Rom edition (2001), CRC Press-Parthenon Publishers, ISBN: 185070368X,
http://www.amazon.com/exec/obidos/ASIN/185070368X/icongroupinter
na

- **Dorland's Illustrated Medical Dictionary (Standard Version)** by Dorland, et al, Hardcover - 2088 pages, 29th edition (2000), W B Saunders Co, ISBN: 0721662544,
http://www.amazon.com/exec/obidos/ASIN/0721662544/icongroupinter
na

- **Dorland's Electronic Medical Dictionary** by Dorland, et al, Software, 29th Book & CD-Rom edition (2000), Harcourt Health Sciences, ISBN: 0721694934,
http://www.amazon.com/exec/obidos/ASIN/0721694934/icongroupinter
na

- **Dorland's Pocket Medical Dictionary (Dorland's Pocket Medical Dictionary, 26th Ed)** Hardcover - 912 pages, 26th edition (2001), W B Saunders Co, ISBN: 0721682812,
http://www.amazon.com/exec/obidos/ASIN/0721682812/icongroupinter
na/103-4193558-7304618

- **Melloni's Illustrated Medical Dictionary (Melloni's Illustrated Medical Dictionary, 4th Ed)** by Melloni, Hardcover, 4th edition (2001), CRC Press-Parthenon Publishers, ISBN: 85070094X,
http://www.amazon.com/exec/obidos/ASIN/85070094X/icongroupintern
a

- **Stedman's Electronic Medical Dictionary Version 5.0 (CD-ROM for Windows and Macintosh, Individual)** by Stedmans, CD-ROM edition (2000), Lippincott Williams & Wilkins Publishers, ISBN: 0781726328,
http://www.amazon.com/exec/obidos/ASIN/0781726328/icongroupinter
na

- **Stedman's Medical Dictionary** by Thomas Lathrop Stedman, Hardcover - 2098 pages, 27th edition (2000), Lippincott, Williams & Wilkins, ISBN:

068340007X,
http://www.amazon.com/exec/obidos/ASIN/068340007X/icongroupinter na

- **Tabers Cyclopedic Medical Dictionary (Thumb Index)** by Donald Venes (Editor), et al, Hardcover - 2439 pages, 19th edition (2001), F A Davis Co, ISBN: 0803606540,
http://www.amazon.com/exec/obidos/ASIN/0803606540/icongroupinter na

INDEX

A

Agenesis.................................47, 78
Airway 200
Anticonvulsive............................67
Apnea..44
Asynchronous.............................48

B

Branch 22, 135, 166, 213
Breakdown 185

C

Compassionate 132
Consultation.......................ii, iii, 3, 35, 205
Consumption 152, 174
Contraindications.............. ii, 133
Cortisol.......................47, 51, 155

D

Deletion......................................70
Discrete 41
Discrimination 41

E

Endorphin 56
Epilepticus................54, 184, 186, 195, 196
Excitability...................40, 46, 155
Excitotoxicity.............................40

F

Fatigue 185
Fetoprotein 193, 210
Fold...196
Fossa..80

G

Growth...............89, 150, 151, 152, 190

H

Handicap 210
Harmony 139
Hereditary 176, 193, 198
Homeobox....................................68
Host...41

I

Impairment 11, 15, 41, 42, 54, 170, 180, 191, 196, 211
Infancy 10, 49, 178
Isoenzyme....................................71

J

Joint 43

L

Linkage 53, 96, 205

M

Medial.................................38, 41
Migration 172
Miscarriage 194
Modeling....................................90
Monoamine................................52
Morphological 62

N

Narcolepsy 175, 180, 181
Need .2, 5, 17, 18, 26, 30, 106, 122, 132, 176, 177, 180, 183, 185, 186, 190, 193, 194, 203
Nerve..........98, 169, 171, 189, 197, 201, 212
Networks..............................3, 42
Nuclei 41, 42

O

Outpatient.................................190

P

Palsy...................... 11, 41, 47, 173
Papilloma 52
Phenotypes 68
Potassium...................................152
Protocol 24

R

Race.................................. 25, 211
Restoration......................139, 140

S

Schizophrenia 42
Segmental................................. 62
Specialist 18
Spectroscopic............................38
Sperm..152

T

Temporal.....38, 41, 43, 77, 97, 177, 188, 210
Thalamic.................................... 63
Therapeutics 131
Threshold 98, 172, 210, 213
Translocation 56
Trauma 171, 183, 196
Tuberous 39, 42, 49, 68, 72, 83, 95, 173

U

Ulcer 55

W

Womb..194
Wound.......................................213

218 Infantile Spasms

780497009854

Printed in the United States
150867LV00009BB/14/A